HEALERS ON HORSEBACK

Other books by the same author ...
> *Animal Psychology*
> *How Animals Talk*
> *The Mind of the Dog*
> *What Makes a Good Horse*
> *The Conformation of the Dog*
> *Veterinary Ophthalmology*
> *Animal Vision*
> *Clinical Veterinary Surgery*
> *The Examination of Animals for Soundness*
> *The Female of the Species*
> *The Anatomy of Dog Breeding*
> *Animal Habits — The Things Animals Do*

HEALERS ON HORSEBACK

The Reminiscences of an English Veterinary Surgeon

By

R. H. SMYTHE, M.R.C.V.S.

Formerly, Examiner for the Diploma of Membership of The Royal College of Veterinary Surgeons

J. A. ALLEN : LONDON

British Library Cataloguing in Publication Data
Smythe, Reginald Harrison
    Healers on Horseback.
        1. Veterinary medicine—England-Cornwall.
        1. Title.
        636.089'092'4   SF658.C/   77-30338
    ISBN 0-85131-282-9

First published 1960, reprinted 1977.

First paperback edition published 1977 by
J. A. Allen & Company Limited,
1 Lower Grosvenor Place, Buckingham Palace Road,
London, SW1W 0EL.

© R. H. Smythe, 1977.

No part of this book may be reproduced or transmitted in any form or by any means, electronic or mechanical, including photocopy, recording, or any information storage and retrieval system now known or to be invented, without permission in writing from the publisher, except by a reviewer who wishes to quote brief passages in connection with a review written for inclusion in a magazine, newspaper or broadcast.

Printed in Great Britain by
Biddles Ltd, Martyr Road, Guildford, Surrey.

FOREWORD

by Brigadier John Clabby, C.B.E., M.R.C.V.S.

R. H. Smythe qualified as a veterinary surgeon at the beginning of this century, now in his ninetieth year he must surely be the doyen of the profession. He gained his working experience at a time when the diagnosis, control and treatment of disease was steadily becoming more scientific and exact. As he indicates, it was a vastly exciting period for the dedicated forward-looking professional man, nevertheless there are still gaps in our knowledge and sometimes useful lessons can be learnt from looking back to the old animal husbandry systems and the manner in which disease problems once were handled.

Reading through this book, which Smythe wrote and had published in 1960, with its nostalgic memories of the unspoiled English countryside, mercifully free of cars and tractors, as it existed 70 years ago, is something of an education. We have forgotten perhaps how much people then relied on their horses and cattle, how closely they linked their lives with them and how well they understood their nature. Only a few skilled stockmen and horsemen now retain this instinctive knowledge of animal behaviour. Not that it was always used for legitimate purposes: the chapter on horse-coping practices leaves one in no doubt that there were rogues around even in those days.

Veterinary medicine itself was at an immature stage and little was known of many diseases. For instance, the metabolic disorders were a complete mystery and milk fever, now easily cured, was a major contributor to the mortality rate among dairy cattle. Inevitably, farmers had their own peculiar remedies for these and other, stranger, diseases such as "worm in the tail" or "bladder under the tongue"; and were apt to blame the evil eye when beset by abortion storms or other calamitous happenings among their stock and so to turn for help to the local wise woman rather than to their veterinary surgeon.

Nevertheless, some of the old remedies are of more than historical interest: after all cures were effected before the advent of antibiotics, and we may wonder with the author whether it is sensible to disregard so completely some of the prescriptions which once apparently served their purpose very well; though cynics may say that the old-style pharmacy, with its pervasive odour of drugs and spices, its huge Latin-labelled jars and bottles, worked a certain magic of its own by inspiring owners with a spurious confidence in the medicines dispensed there.

The author describes this other world with wit and charm, and with some regret for its passing. But there is no lack of enthusiasm either for the modern developments in veterinary medicine and surgery; or for the successful campaigns leading to the elimination of bovine tuberculosis and other scourges that once posed a threat to animal health, and very often to human health as well.

However, he is far from complacent and in his final chapter he makes thoughtful comment on the measures still needed to improve the lot of our horses, pets and farm animals which play such an important part in our lives. Though written some years ago these suggestions are worth pondering on today.

JOHN CLABBY
1977

CONTENTS

	Page
FOREWORD	v

Chapter One. A LONG WHILE AGO 3
Attitude towards animals—The old way and the new—The mechanistic outlook—The veterinary environment—Blood sports—Pharmacy then and now—Modern drugs—The drug trade is Big Business—Wild goats and tame ones—The goat and the wrestler—Goat Editor—How to milk a goat—Cattle in Cornwall—Cattle as pets—Fetch the veterinary—Client appreciation—The client-practitioner relationship—The Survey Scheme—Horse breeding—Local rodeo—The branding—Wild ponies—Hunting was popular—Colt-breaking—Horse dealing—Horses were essential—The advent of the motor car—Women veterinary surgeons—A carter's day—Prestige of the horseman—A story of devotion—Our dependence on the horse—Saddle versus buggy—Riding on the roof—Jockey's neck.

Chapter Two. THE FIRST FORTY YEARS ARE THE HARDEST 19
Progress of science—The old remedies are no more—The new ones come and go—The remedy or the disease—Did the old practitioners do any good?—Enthusiasm and disappointment—A tradition to maintain—Spadework and prestige—Why we practise—Endurance test—Asleep in the saddle—The doctor and the veterinary shared their common lot—Women on the doorstep—Hoof beats by night—The night bell—Nocturnal farming—The witching hour—The advent of the phone—Night work—Calving—Horse or car—Doing thirty—Competition rears its head—Hospitals—The influence of motordom—Witchcraft at work—Witch versus witch—Getting rid of the enemy—Charlatans of today—

Psychological treatment—Surgery ancient and modern—Physiology—Choice of profession—A change of background—Animal interests—Animal Husbandry and Animal Management—No hospital wards—Extra-mural tuition—At home with animals—Country doctor—Small animal practice—The eminence of modern veterinary science—The economical handicap—Cost of animal treatment—Specialisation—Laboratory work—Animal Health Division—General practice—Research—Composite practices.

Chapter Three. SETTING-UP IN PRACTICE 38
Illusion and fact—The gift of martyrdom—Learning the hard way—Medical examination—Stresses and the endocrine system—Introverts and extroverts—A leaning towards celibacy— Partnership—The bedside manner—Putting up a plate—The ethical code—Quacks—Caesarian operation—Mining—Increase in population—Educating the client—Value for money—Cattle and ironmongery—The post-mortem—The knacker—A little bit of luck.

Chapter Four. SOME DISEASES OF ANIMALS 48
Milk fever or hypocalcaemia—The old treatment and the new—The whiskey remedy—Hypomagnesaemia—The ghost cow—Tubercle and Johne's disease—The Tuberculosis Order—Elimination of the disease—Raw milk—Children and tubercle—A matter of warranty—Indigestion—Acetonaemia—Recent advances in cattle practice—The dutiful Billy goat—Contagious abortion and undulant fever—An exaggerated prognosis—Psittacosis and ornithosis—Pasteuration and sterilisation of milk—Animals in captivity—Simian virus B—Poliomyelitis vaccine—Notifiable diseases—Preventive medicine—Meat inspection—Veterinary pathology.

Chapter Five. HORSE PRACTICE 67
Examination for soundness—Dealer's tricks—Never on Sunday—Holding-up the traffic—Docking—On the village green—Cornish donkeys—Chariot racing—A yardful of horses—Physiotherapy—

Page

Thermo-cautery—Low-wave therapy—Infectious diseases—Bowel derangements—Monday morning legs—Ophthalmia—Haemoglobinuria—The old grey mare—Castration—Risks to the operator The boar pig—A veterinary hospital—Equine surgery.

Chapter Six. SMALL ANIMAL PRACTICE 85
Neurotic dogs and anxious owners—The embarrassing female—Foreign bodies—Fish hooks and rubber bones—Other bones—Nylons—Eye diseases and heredity—Short lived spines—Nephritis—Leptospiral jaundice—Virus diseases—X-ray examination—Cataract operations and corneal grafting—Urine testing—Dog breeders—Business or hobby—Spirit of competition—Dogs on honeymoon—Pink noses—Man and dog in partnership—Guard dogs—Lost dog—Euthanasia—The G.I.'s and the Dane—A resurrection.

Chapter Seven. VETERINARY OBSTETRICS 100
This craze for Caesarian operations—Infertility—Artificial insemination—Seeing practice—A dominant female—Calving routine—A shortage of soap—A delayed departure—A matter of nationality—Anaesthesia—Disappearing helpers—Obstetrics in comfort—A duel in the cowshed—Daniel—The provisions of Nature.

Chapter Eight. THE DIFFICULTY OF BEING A VETERINARY SURGEON . 116
Doctors and veterinary surgeons—Animals do not talk—On being animal-minded—The modern background—Women have keener perception—The craving for speed and space—A new way of life—On being successful—Clinical observation—Surgical asepsis—Antibiotics—Bowel resection—Something missing—A bath in the parlour—The bed warmer—Lost dog—Down the shaft—An expensive guest.

Chapter Nine. WHAT OF THE FUTURE? 127
Animals and our national economy—Animals for food—Human enterprise—Our national food supply—Animals and our own

psychology—Animals as a safety valve—Animals in sport—The Royal College of Veterinary Surgeons—The British Veterinary Association—The Universities—Extra-mural tuition—Economics—Charitable institutions—Overheads—Meat inspection—Client relationship—Combined practice—Nationalisation—Veterinary hospitals—Maintaining our prestige.

HEALERS ON HORSEBACK

Chapter One

A LONG WHILE AGO

It would be difficult to say when first I started to work in a veterinary practice, for I was born in one.

All my spare time when I was not in school, every half-day, and weekend, was spent travelling around with my father while he visited farms and stables. When we did not ride side by side, we journeyed together behind a horse in a two-wheeled buggy.

Arrived at our destination I was kept busy running backwards and forwards from and to this vehicle, fetching the various appliances, instruments or drugs as they were wanted for each patient. I helped to handle the animals, to soothe the horses with my voice, and to scruff the less amenable cattle by nose and horns—and woe betide me if ever I let go!

Occasionally we visited dogs, but all this happened well over sixty years ago, when canine practice had not attained the importance with which it is regarded today by practitioners and clients alike.

As we travelled along the country roads from one farm to another, my father would talk to me about the case he had last dealt with, ask me what I had observed, and explain to me all the items I had overlooked.

I thought then—and I still think—my father was a wonderful man, very observant and a true clinician, but I fear that in the opinion of the young graduate, fresh today from his University training, he would have been considered woefully ignorant since he would have lacked the modern teachings associated with the subjects of physiology, pathology and bacteriology. Our modern graduates would have been in a similar position, of course, if the practitioners of earlier generations had not worked hard and acquired the knowledge which has been handed down to *this* generation. It will now be the turn of the young people to acquire more and more learning and pass it on to *their* children and grandchildren.

But the modern graduates would not have gained all the marks. My father had been reared and educated in a world very different from the one they inhabit. He had lived always among animals. He probably knew a great deal more about their anatomy than the present generation of veterinary surgeons are likely to do, and he certainly knew a great deal more about the animals themselves; about animals as individuals, and about their needs; what made them comfortable and happy; what they liked and what they disliked—in modern phraseology, "how they ticked."

He lived much closer to the animal mind than modern youth could approach, or would ever wish to. Animals were as near and dear to my father as his own children and I, as one of the latter, respected him for it.

He was not alone in this respect for his fellow practitioners were all moulded on the same plan. In company with all of these, my father at that time had never yet driven a mechanically-propelled vehicle, but from his childhood he had ridden and driven every kind of horse, had probably milked every kind of cow, and had hunted with, or shot over, every kind of hound and gundog.

He regarded his patients as living flesh and blood, each entitled to a place in a communal world, endowed with needs and emotions all their own.

In these mechanatomic days there is an ever-growing tendency to regard the animal as being built in sections, to regard each anatomical system as a unit, in much the same way as the motorist looks upon a carburettor, a petrol pump, or upon some appliance adapted to ridding the machine of its chemical exhaust.

It is a common failing to imagine that animal tissues, energised by blood and activated by nervous impulses, can be expected to function with the same degree of exactitude demanded of mechanical appliances constructed from metal. This may be partly because modern practitioners are so dependent upon mechanised power that their own minds tend to operate mechanically. Life today encourages the mechanistic outlook.

I recall that during my schooldays and at sixteen years of age when I left school to prepare for my four years at College (the period has increased considerably now), my whole interest in life was closely linked up with animals, and since I had been raised in a veterinary environment I was particularly concerned with animal health and disease, with prophylaxis and treatment.

But in those days, hard as we worked, we managed to get some time free to indulge in our hobbies. When quite a child I contrived to get together a vast and weird collection of animals of many kinds, and from my early years, or as soon as I could climb onto a horse, my hours of freedom were devoted to hunting, shooting and fishing.

Although I must confess that age has lessened by enthusiasm regarding the so-called "blood sports," and made me very unwilling to cause unnecessary suffering to any living creature, I am the first to realise and to admit that my change of feeling is due solely to failure of my endocrine system to produce the requisite supply of hormones, and is in no way the result of acquired virtue.

When my blood was hot and youthful, I was as eager to kill as other young people are today.

When we encounter folk who vehemently demand the immediate abolition of amusements obtained at the expense of any animal, who scream for an end to be put to hunting, fishing, fly swatting, shooting and other sportsmanlike pastimes, we can depend upon it that they were pampered in their youth, lacked opportunity to kill while their blood was young and their natural instincts uninhibited; or they are old fogeys, like myself, who have outlived their lust for excitement and are now flat out, seeking absolution for the sins of their youth.

As a youngster attending a local grammar school, I used to spend a lot of my time, particularly when the weather was too wet to enable me to indulge in a spot of poaching, hard at work in my father's dispensary, pounding up vast quantities of carbonate of ammonia, all in huge lumps, like and nearly as hard as rocks, mixing the resulting powder with sacksful of gentian and foenugrec, aniseed and ginger, and packing the mixture up into four ounce parcels, hundreds of them, each one neatly wrapped in brown paper and sealed with wax. Or, I would stand watching jars of aloes set up in a water bath over a lighted gas ring, awaiting the critical moment when the contents would attain the correct consistence without the water, below and around the jar, ever coming to the boil; and I would spend hours rolling and wrapping the resulting confection into "horse balls," resembling three inch lengths cut off a mahogany walking stick. Each one of these had to be wrapped neatly in thin white paper, and later on I would be privileged occasionally to peel off my jacket, roll up my sleeves and push some of these balls down the throats of unwilling horses. On another afternoon I would be mixing the embrocation—the "horse oils"—shaking the heavy winchesters until their contents emulsified, filling innumerable eight ounce bottles with the creamy fluid, corking and labelling them ready for use.

Or it might be pint-and-a-half bottles of cattle drenches, six doses in each, containing a wonderful assortment of drugs, each bottle labelled with a red warning notice forbidding the farmer to hold the cow's head above the level of her body and advising him to make sure that she swallowed one mouthful safely before he administered the next.

The black draughts for the relief of colic were great favourites of mine, not because I suffered from any digestive aberration, but because I was permitted to cut their corks level with the neck of the bottle and dip each bottle, held upside down, into a saucepan containing an inch of boiling pitch.

In those days pharmacy was an art which nowadays is completely neglected, seldom taught.

My father's dispensary, in spite of the vast amount of work which went on within it, had to be kept dustless and shining. The large benches of old mahogany, black with age, must be polished each evening with beeswax and turpentine (also prepared on the premises) and heaven help the sinner who left even a measure glass an inch out of its recognised position.

I often wonder what would be the reactions of a modern University student if he, or she, were suddenly transported back to the "good old days" when one shut doors softly, kept premises and selves spotlessly tidy, and were presented with a granite mortar and a heavy marble pestle, and required to reduce a quarter of a hundred-weight of rock-hard ammonium carbonate to a fine powder which would all pass through a hair sieve.

Today, the drugs of the British Pharmacopoeia repose, despised and neglected, in the cellars of the wholesale druggists. Few students know them even by name, and the majority are quite ignorant regarding their dosage.

Instead, our modern graduates act nowadays as distribution agents for scores of drug houses, doling out to their clients attractive little packages of antibiotics, vermicides, hormones, flea killers, and a variety of other new medicaments, the contents of which they may never have seen, depending entirely upon the pseudo-scientific jargon issued with each packet by the pharmaceutical firm which supplies them. It is not the veterinary surgeon alone who avails himself of this easy, but expensive, method of prescribing. Now that the old recognised remedies have been discarded and dispensing is a thing of the past, the sister professions of human and veterinary medicine are equally concerned in this wholesale distribution of specifics for every known and unknown complaint.

And yet I look back upon those far-off days, and nights, armed with the pestle and the pill-roller, with feelings of nostalgia. They were undoubtedly the happiest days of my life, shared with equally happy and wonderfully pleasant companions.

The days of the angry young men were still a long way ahead. I suppose away back in those times we young people were not very bright, a fact which accounted for our contentment.

I well remember when I first entered the Royal Veterinary College, being taken to London, in company with another seventeen-year-old lad who was to share rooms with me, by my father and mother, who were careful that the two of us should not get into bad company. I remember, too, embarking on an expedition around Camden Town where they proposed to find us suitable "digs." We went into dozens of houses which were not to my parents' liking, and we were eventually deposited, trunks and all, in a house which within a few hours of my parents' departure quickly demonstrated itself to be a brothel, and one of doubtful vintage at that. Returning from College the following evening I found that my box had been rifled and the three months allowance given me all in one sum, in order that it might encourage a sense of responsibility, was missing.

We were eventually seen off the premises by a constable, who appeared biased in favour of our landladies; but that is quite another story. The point was that in order to hide my loss and struggle through my first three months at College, I started to write, and quite naturally I made animals my main topic. It commenced this way:

Before I left home I had been investigating the behaviour of a herd of wild goats which roamed the North Cliffs of Cornwall. The Billy of the herd was something of a humorist. He would sight a courting couple seated on the cliff edge with their feet dangling over a three-hundred-foot precipice, and would then approach very quietly from behind, give a huge snort and announce his proximity. Various tales were told about what Billy did next, but the only authentic account was of one occasion on which a celebrated Cornish wrestler took his girl friend onto the cliffs. The last account of either Billy or the wrestler, given by his girl friend, was that the wrestler, when last seen, was holding Billy by its horns afraid to let go, and Billy was standing his ground firmly and prepared to do so for a week, awaiting his chance to propel the wrestler bodily over the cliffs. I understood that the young lady, becoming bored with the spectacle, walked quietly home and left the pair to work out their own problem.

I sent this story to a popular journal and made enough out of it to pay the rent of my new digs for a week, and in the nick of time I received an invitation from a well-known paper to write them an article on goats. The Editor wanted particularly to hear whether I really knew a great deal about these animals. At that time I did not, but I refrained from admitting it, and from a little judicious correspondence I discovered that nobody on the staff of the paper knew anything either, so I took a chance. As a result I was promptly appointed Goat Editor, with a weekly column to write. At seventeen this was fame indeed although, of course, the Editor of the paper had no idea of my youthfulness as our business had been all transacted by correspondence.

My first procedure was to purchase a nicely illustrated book from which I discovered that married lady goats carried very large udders and that their teats almost touched the ground. It was obvious to me that such an animal must require very tactful milking, especially if one suffered from twinges of lumbago. I decided, therefore, to start right by contributing a column on "How to Milk a Goat."

Never having seen this operation performed made it a little more difficult, and I worked it out on the lines that if Mahomet could not be persuaded to come to the mountain, then the mountain must come to Mahomet. Or, so I reasoned.

In the end I drew a Heath Robinson type of illustration for my article, in which the lady goat, bribed by the offer of luscious carrots, was persuaded to walk up an inclined gangway, something like that by which one enters a liner. At the top she stood upon a board, with her head held firmly by a trevis which dropped over her neck, like the old-fashioned stocks in the market place. Now comes the clever part of the idea. While the lady was regaling herself on the bunch of carrots dangled in front of her nose, a trapdoor opened immediately below her udder, and in my illustration the proud owner, still in his city tails and striped trousers, stood and milked her into a pail hung at a suitable distance below her.

The editor of the paper took the idea quite seriously; a firm specializing in such ingenious appliances commenced to manufacture it without conferring with its inventor, and a milking platform on similar lines may be seen in use even today in many of the most up-to-date goat farms.

I tell this story simply to excuse myself for writing at all, since without that goat I should never have written the article or become goat editor, and I should never have struggled through that first three months, eventually to become a veterinary surgeon, in fact I might never have entered the profession at all.

Veterinary practice in England, sixty years ago, was quite unlike what it is today.

In Cornwall, in which county my father carried on a very extensive practice, the farms were usually small but very heavily stocked. The number of dairy cattle in the county was fantastic and it was estimated that the circumscribed area my father served, roughly 120 square miles, carried 28,000 cows, mostly Guernseys with some Jerseys and a few Shorthorns. Friesians had not at that time arrived in any number. There were also a good many South Devons used mainly for beef production, and where these existed in numbers the percentage of Guernseys was lower.

At that time the cattle population was so great that it used to be said locally that if the total increased by another 1 per cent, then several hundred cattle stood a risk of being pushed over the edges of the Cornish cliffs. As many of these were 300 feet high, it could truthfully be said that the cattle population had reached its economic limit.

From the veterinary aspect Cornwall was a paradise, since the cattle were petted and treated as members of the family, and the veterinary surgeon was regarded as the most important member of the community.

Because they were so well cared for, it was not uncommon for Guernsey cows to rear fourteen successive calves and then to become pensioners until they died of old age. The economic disadvantages of this type of farming never impressed itself on the Cornish farmer who would as soon think of murdering his grandmother as sending Tremayne's Dolores VIII to the knacker just because she had outlived her period of service.

If the least thing went wrong with a cow, a calf or a bull; if it coughed twice in a morning, was a wee bit loose in its motions, or slightly lame, and especially if a cow showed any udder or teat abnormality, the veterinary surgeon was summoned post-haste, and all the family from near and far and a goodly collection of the neighbours, would be grouped on the spot to meet him and hear his opinion regarding the suffering animal.

At calving-time each Guernsey received as much attention as an expectant princess and the veterinary surgeon would be required to make ante-natal examinations, and asked to give the cow a "lookover" about the expected date of her calving "just to be on the safe side."

It was not unusual for these high-yielding cows to show signs of impending milk fever (hypocalcaemia) two or three days before calving, in which case, after the discovery of the advantages of calcium therapy, they received hypodermic injections of calcium borogluconate at intervals until the third day after calving. If a cow went a day or two past her time the whole village knew it and she would become the main topic of conversation in the village "local," where bets might be made on the sex of the calf and the time of its birth.

This awareness and appreciation of the value of veterinary service, and a complete dependence upon professional skill, was widespread throughout the county and the client-practitioner relationship was much closer than I have seen it in any other part of the country.

In one or two districts where beef cattle were more extensively bred the economic situation was regarded as being more important, and sentiment was less obvious. Farmers, in these circumstances were inclined sometimes to fall into the clutches of the patent medicine vendors, usually with disastrous results and a rapid return to the veterinary fold.

This striking difference between the farmers of the Cornish peninsula and those of the rest of the country was manifested very clearly during the Second World War, when the Survey Scheme was devised with the object of getting the veterinary surgeon onto the farm and allowing the British public to benefit from the increased production of food stuffs and dairy produce, which it was believed would ensue as a result of veterinary advice. It was also the intention to cull animals which were not producing calves and milk and replace they by others that would do so.

Undoubtedly, over large areas of the country the Survey Scheme served a very useful purpose but the Cornish veterinary surgeons decided that what *they* needed was not a means of getting onto the farm but an opportunity to get *off* farms where they were not so urgently required in order that they might devote more time to farms where their help would be of vital importance. So firm was their belief in their clients, and in the degree of confidence in their services repeatedly expressed by the farmers, that the numerous firms of veterinary surgeons in the county stood out from the Scheme and carried on as they had always done. I do not think that the committee sponsoring the scheme ever fully understood the Cornish situation, or ever realized that Cornwall was the one county in England in which the farmers made completely sure at all times that their cattle received veterinary attention on the slightest provocation.

Horse breeding, sixty years ago, was at its highest level throughout the British Isles, both as regards the number of foals produced annually and the outstanding quality of British horses. We had every kind of horse, Thoroughbreds, hunters, hackneys, hacks and cobs, with Shire horses, Clydesdales and Suffolk Punches in great numbers.

Horse practice was at its best. In addition the moors, including Dartmoor, Exmoor, the New Forest, the Highlands of Scotland and the Welsh hills and mountains, all carried large droves of wild or semi-wild ponies.

Every year these ponies had to be rounded up, and branded, the entires picked out and all the surplus males castrated. Annual sales were the rule, and these were often coupled with an amateur rodeo in which the village lads tried out their skill on bareback, buckjumping ponies. Every village had its fairs and sales and to see the streets thronged with ponies and farmers was a remarkable sight.

The urgent need to castrate all these colts cast a springtime burden upon the already over-employed veterinary surgeons.

The Dartmoor ponies, additional to the normal colt production on every farm, were our main concern during a restricted period. These colts were not large, but when one tried to handle them they appeared to possess all the slipperiness of an eel with a similar capacity for tying themselves in knots. One could imagine that they possessed more than the usual allowance of four limbs with which to lash out in all directions, and these limbs and feet potentially were very dangerous weapons.

The grown stallions, too, had an unpleasant way of standing straight up on their hind limbs and feet, manipulating their fore feet after the style of a boxer and would march down, upon and over anyone who happened to make the least attempt to obstruct their passage. It was virtually impossible to put halters on these unbroken ponies and it usually came to lassooing them, using a rope which would not draw the loop sufficiently tight to cause suffocation.

Any veterinary surgeon who could catch, cast and castrate a score of such animals in the better part of a day, and return home unscathed, usually regarded himself as being particularly fortunate.

Hunting in those days, far more so than at present, was one of the great interests of the countryside. Hounds were welcomed by the farmers and convenient gates were left open, while wire was rarely used.

Nearly every farmer bred a few hunter foals every year, usually by a Thoroughbred stallion out of a Shire or half-bred mare, and in due course broke and trained them himself, or with the help of a colt-breaker.

Colt-breaking was a recognised trade and a man who had four or five hunter colts in hand at all times and was paid to stable and feed them, too, was doing quite well for himself. As soon as they could be safely ridden in company, the farmer, or his son, usually hunted them regularly with the local pack of foxhounds, until somebody took a fancy to one of them and purchased it. A good four-year-old fetched a lot of money, even so long ago, and although it might have paid better to feed a cow than a couple of colts, the sporting instincts of the farmer and his family were gratified, and combining business with pleasure in the hunting field considerably relieved the monotony of life. Occasionally some "foreign" millionaire, that is to say one hailing from north of the river Tamar, would tour the country, picking up a few good hunters for himself and his friends. The Cornish were very honest people among themselves. It has often been asserted that dealing in any shape or form arouses man's baser instincts, and I have an uncomfortable suspicion that the conspiracy among these Cornish farmers, designed to "take a rise out of the foreigner" was often only too well organised.

A great many Shire foals were also raised from working mares and the majority of these were kept for work on the farm, or sold to brewery firms and other trades when old enough to work on the roads. These were as essential for farm work and transport as the lorries and tractors of modern times.

It must be hard for young people today to picture the roads of only a few decades ago when horses were everywhere, and the motor car was famous more on account of its nuisance value than its utility.

The sudden rise of motor transport hit the horse trade very badly and it was feared that its effect upon veterinary practice would be disastrous. But, as must always happen, and may yet do again, the profession found another outlet, or several in fact.

One of these was additional employment as local veterinary surgeons to the Ministry of Agriculture; another was the extension of canine and small animal practice.

The latter brought a large number of women into the profession. They enlisted ostensibly for small animal work but the shortage of veterinary surgeons throughout the country, soon enabled them to undertake general practice, when it was found they were equally as efficient in treating large animals as small. At first the farming fraternity were a little diffident regarding women practitioners on the farms but since those early days women veterinary surgeons have proved remarkably successful and they now hold important positions, in practice, as research workers and as teachers in the universities, which they adorn with their presence, while their superlative ability has led to a universal appreciation of their value to the community.

While horses were employed almost wholly on the farms, and for road haulage, horsemen were always in great demand. A good carter who took pride in his horses, would care for his tackle and be hard at work from 5 a.m. until his final round of inspection at 9 p.m., and was willing to be on call seven days a week, held a high place in the esteem of his employer. The degree of prestige attached to a good horseman was much higher than is today afforded to the best tractor hands and lorry drivers.

The horseman was singled out as an individual, and it took a long apprenticeship to enable him to thoroughly understand horses and their requirements. Moreover, horses coming in wet and mud-stained from work needed cleaning and attention before they could be left. Their wants could not be satisfied by the turn of an ignition key. The farm carter was a man for whom I always entertained the highest regard. They have now died out and their kind exists no longer. Their grandchildren, like the vehicles they drive, have become completely mechanised.

I would like to relate an incident which will better illustrate the devotion which the simple farm carter lavished on his horses:

It concerns a horseman of the old school, who lived in a farm cottage almost opposite the stables. His favourite mare was very ill and I diagnosed a torsion of the large intestine with an undoubtedly fatal prognosis.

It would have been much kinder to have carried out euthanasia and put the poor animal out of her misery, but John, the carter, would have believed ever after that the mare might have recovered.

All I could do was keep her mercifully under the influence of morphia and chloral until her end came.

I saw the mare first on a Monday evening. John nursed her continuously with the full knowledge that in the "vet's" opinion nothing could save her. I paid them both a visit every few hours during night and day, until the Thursday morning when the mare died. Never for a single moment had John left his patient during all those days and nights.

Such devotion to an animal was most touching.

John shed a tear or two, dashing them from his eyes with his knuckles as though ashamed of his weakness. As the mare kicked her way out of life, lying on her side on the ground, he sat on a stool with his head bowed and hidden in the sleeve of his greatcoat.

Presently he looked up and said to me: "Well, the old girl's gone now. You're certain you couldn't have done nothing more for her?"

"No," I assured him. "You haven't anything to blame yourself for; I think you've been wonderful."

"It's right glad I be to hear 'ee say so," he replied. "I suppose I'd better be away across and take a look at the missus now. She was confined last Tuesday."

During my early days in veterinary practice we depended in rural districts entirely upon the horse as our method of transport, unless we could ride bicycles. In those days bicycles were not so comfortable as today, and metalled roads in many parts of the country were almost non-existent.

On any occasion on which we were compelled to carry a good deal of tackle for casting animals, stocks of medicine and instruments, we found it easier to load all these things into the boot of the buggy.

A four-wheeled "wagonette" with a closed "dickey" at the rear was ideal, but being heavy it required a big horse, while for a buggy a 14.3 h.h. cob was very suitable.

In spite of the advantages and indeed the luxury of driving round the countryside, sitting on a cushioned seat with a waterproof rug tucked warmly around the knees, all dressed up in a waterproof coat and a Sou'Wester hat, we yet found that for short rounds and emergency calls the saddle horse was quicker and far less trouble as there was no muddy buggy to wash on returning home, and no wet harness to be cleaned. Certainly, we usually kept a groom and a stable lad, but scraping thick mud off wheels and polishing a trap twice daily was not their idea of enjoyment either.

One could so easily ride a horse across country from farm to farm. One soon learned the whereabouts of gaps and which were the lowest banks. Fortunately wire was not popular in that hunting country and electric fences had not been invented.

I have vivid recollections of visiting a farm in the wildest part of Cornwall. I was on horseback and I was riding in company with some other people who were visiting the same premises for which I was bound, it being the occasion of a farm sale.

One of my companions was the auctioneer and two more were dealers.

None of us had any detailed knowledge of this part of the country, but one of the dealers pretended that he had, and so he led the party. His name was Frank Newman, and under his guidance everything at first went well. We rode across a moor, jumping a few low stone walls built up from granite boulders, went over a dyke or two, then pulled up at what at first appeared to be a high Cornish bank, almost impossible to jump. It was at least seven feet high and very solid in appearance.

The party came to a halt.

Frank Newman and myself were mounted on Cornish-bred cobs about 14.3 h.h. while the others rode hunters of considerable size and substance.

Frank was a fine horseman and his Cherry and my Tim had often raced side-by-side and hunted together, so where one went the other would surely follow. Cherry had won a good many point-to-points in spite of her small size.

"I'll show you the way over," shouted Frank with a laugh.

It was not at all ambitious but I had little choice. These Cornish cobs were remarkable jumpers and having been used all their lives to earthen banks, had learned that the highest of them could be conquered by a combination of jumping so far and climbing the rest. Coming down off the other side was simple, depending only upon the inexorable laws of gravity.

Before I realised what was happening Cherry was climbing onto the top of that enormous bank and I, on Tim, was fast approaching its foot.

Cherry having reached the top, stood precariously balanced there, looking down on the other side with a decidedly surprised look, even for a Cornish cob to wear on her face. By this time Tim was up there beside her and I could swear that they cocked an eye at each other as they surveyed the scene below.

From the top of the bank to the ground would have been a simple jump of about nine feet, but there was something in the way. Right along that bank, three feet from its top, there stretched the lean-to galvanised roof of a range of piggeries. The roof sloped sharply downwards to a front elevation of only six feet.

To this day I thank my lucky stars that the roof was of high quality and brand new, for with a clatter that could have been heard for miles the two cobs jumped together onto the top of that metal roof, sat on their sterns, and slid down to the lower edge, pitched off and landed on all four feet, arriving without mark or injury, and quite ready to go on their way as if tobaggoning off tin roofs was part of their ordinary routine.

What would have happened if that roof had been thin and rusty, I dread to think.

I mention this little incident to illustrate the fact that although riding on horseback had many advantages, it was not entirely devoid of excitement, but it did enable one to reach places where no buggy could penetrate.

This applied particularly to hill farms, often approachable after travelling along narrow tracks between granite boulders, safely negotiable only by a pony or a goat.

When first I went to school as a five-year-old, I used to spend my Wednesday and Saturday afternoons visiting farms with my father, when they were not too far from home.

I would be mounted on one of my young donkeys and my father would ride Stella, a thoroughbred mare.

As a child, I used to invest my pocket money in donkeys. I could buy young ones at from half-a-sovereign to a sovereign apiece, break them in and sell them later for several pounds, buying fresh ones in their place.

Stella would knock along at a fast trot and the donkey would canter or gallop, trying to keep a couple of paces ahead of her. But when Stella put on a spurt and drew level with the donkey, the latter would invariably plant both fore feet firmly on the ground and come to an abrupt halt.

Each time this happened, I would shoot feet over the donkey's head, usually landing upon my own.

This would happen several times on each trip.

A great many years later, when I was x-rayed following an accident, the radiologist reported that the patient showed every indication of possessing a "jockey's neck." This was the first occasion upon which this particular interpretation of an x-ray film had come to my notice, and although between my donkey-riding days and the taking of the x-ray film I had done a lot of cross-country riding, I have very little doubt as to the time of my life during which I did most of that "jockeying."

Chapter Two

THE FIRST FORTY YEARS ARE THE HARDEST

W<small>HEN ONE CASTS</small> the mind back over a mere score of years, one cannot help but be astonished at the discoveries which have been made and the changes which have come to pass during this short period.

Scientific workers make countless discoveries on each successive day. Drug firms need hardly do so; they have already discovered how profitable it is to use one of the discoveries, hash and re-hash it simply by presenting the same product again and again under a different name. Each time the price is a little higher than it was before. The drugs we depended upon as little as a score of years ago have vanished from our shelves. We older folk have watched the arrival of the all-conquering sulfa drugs, the panacea for all ills, the key to life everlasting.

We have seen them on their way out—they have almost vanished already. In their place came penicillin, but the germs learned how to resist its effects and now the fame of this original antibiotic is waning—it had unfortunate side effects in some cases and it engendered allergies in many patients. In its place have rushed—there is no more suitable word—a hundred new antibiotics all eager to show off their paces, and as yet we do not know whether their worst effects will be upon the patient or upon the germs which assail him or her.

One cannot help wondering whether all the efforts of the older practitioners who depended upon the British Pharmacopoeia, were entirely wasted, and if it is true that cures have only been effected since specific antibiotics have come into general use. Have the healing powers of nature departed too, or may they not still occasionally play some small part in bringing about recovery?

Did we older practitioners really do no good in all our years of practice and is this new generation responsible for miracles of healing unheard of in previous history?

Were we old hands only deceiving our clients as well as ourselves, or was the advice we gave even more valuable than our medicines?

History has a habit, too, of repeating itself, and the enthusiasms of yesterday are apt to become the disappointments of tomorrow.

How long, one wonders, will some of our more recent treatments continue in use before someone discovers their dangers, and demonstrates that their side effects and their long-term potentialities make it advisable to take them off the market?

A veterinary surgeon, one of my friends, who had suffered five months agony from a persistent pruritus, the result of being dosed with a new and little known antibiotic for the treatment of some minor ailment, remarked very truthfully that the only people who know a great deal about the effects of modern drugs are the patients to whom they are administered.

Neither the firms who sell them, nor the professional men who prescribe them, can ever sample the lot and judge from first hand experience just what they may do to the patient.

Not every layman, lying awake in bed at night with a persistently itching anus, which is driving him nearly crazy, would associate his present discomfort with the half-dozen capsules of antibiotic he swallowed five weeks ago. If the clinician, medical or veterinary, who departed this life only ten years ago, could return to earth today, he would need to be completely re-educated before becoming sufficiently up-to-date to treat a simple case of acne.

But this is a digression for which I crave forgiveness.

It is probably good sometimes to look back upon the past if one wishes to appreciate the advantages of the present. I can turn back the pages of my own book of life and recollect with thankfulness the hardships experienced during countless days and nights of work as a veterinary surgeon, none of which, in any way similar, are likely to assail the modern graduate.

All of us who embrace an open-air profession (and country practitioners seldom suffer from lack of oxygen), have a great tradition to maintain.

Those who have enjoyed veterinary practice for a mere dozen years, have tasted only its luxury, they have missed those tougher days of experiment and endeavour, when the exercising of the veterinary art was attended by hardship, often accompanied by farmyard squalor. And yet, in spite of all it endured the profession retained and increased its prestige; the practitioner gained the confidence and respect of his clients and held a high place in their affection. It was this preliminary spadework, the hardship and the suffering so cheerfully overcome, which paved the way for a new generation of graduates, and it is the prestige founded by the older generation which they have inherited.

Let us hope that this new generation will rise above becoming mere distributors of other firms' packed goods, that they will learn to use their eyes and employ their senses to diagnose, rather than depend upon physical aids. May they also learn to understand the lives led by normal healthy animals as much as they do those of the sick. Veterinary practice is not only a way of earning a living, it is a vocation to which one is dedicated, by which one strives to provide for the so-called "lower animals" the ministrations which our sister profession provides for more favoured human beings.

Those of us who had fathers engaged in medical or veterinary practice sixty-odd years ago, did not follow in their footsteps merely because we were seeking an easy, care-free existence, nor did we waste a great deal of thought upon the possible size of our bank balance.

We knew where we were heading from the very start. We became doctors because we could at least tolerate humanity and because we disliked watching human suffering unless we were in a position to bring it relief.

We became veterinary surgeons, not because we sought a job with regular hours and the prospect of wealth, but because we liked animals and sympathised with them; also, perhaps, because we experienced a feeling of gladness when we induced animals to like us.

None of us harboured any false conception about the kind of life that lay ahead. We expected to have to make many sacrifices, to work long hours by day and by night as well; to be at everybody's beck and call.

We were ready, eager even, to give service to animals and their owners at all times, for little and often for no pecuniary reward.

None but those who practised fifty or sixty years ago can have the least understanding of what was endured and accepted by doctors and veterinary surgeons alike, as part and parcel of their normal existence.

I need not dwell unduly upon the endless hours spent in the saddle through all hours of the day and night.

Riding on horseback was accepted by all ranks as the orthodox means of travelling from one place to another, irrespective of weather conditions, wealth or rank.

We rode over the hills, the moors and the dales in sunshine, darkness, in hail and rain and snow. We tied sacks around the feet of our horses when the roads were icy, and we walked miles beside them when fog descended on the moors and the bogs lay ready to engulf us.

We carried on frequently for days and nights on horseback without sleep, although some of us could sleep in the saddle without losing our grip. It was by no means rare for a horseman to return homewards asleep, leaving navigation entirely to his horse.

We appreciated fine weather when it came, but just as often we rode along soaked to the skin, so cold we could hardly hold the reins.

But it was rarely one ever heard a complaint from one's fellow companions—it was all in the day's work.

Looking back as I now do, I would hesitate to say that those were my most unhappy days.

I am not trying to give the impression that the country veterinary surgeon was unique in his suffering. The medical practitioner with clients all over the countryside shared our lot and worked under exactly the same conditions.

Neither the "vet" nor the doctor, had learned the habit of self-indulgence. There was little thought of holidays, we had never heard of leisure by rota, the five-day-week, or any of the enticements practitioners now use to bait their supplications whenever they require another assistant.

My own father worked very hard for his first twenty years in practice before he decided he was justified in taking a few days holiday out of sight of his surgery.

In company with all other outdoor workers, professional or otherwise, the men of his day were tough folk, accustomed to living the hard way.

We, and I can include myself among them, agreed with Shakespeare when he wrote:

"For suffering is the badge of all our tribe."

The country doctor and the country veterinary surgeon shared a great deal in common. They met, or passed each other, or rode along side-by-side on their daily rounds. On o. occasions they waved their whips to one another as they went past in their buggies, and neither was accounted a hero by his public simply because he was a weary man lacking time to dry his breeches.

We had no telephones, of course, in those days and between 9 a.m. and 7 p.m. most of our distant calls came by telegram, or by messenger galloping on horseback. When we opened the door of our waiting room every morning at eight o'clock, we would find waiting on the doorstep, a gathering of country women, the wives or servants of the farmers, with requests for visits, or demands for medicine.

Most of them wore hobnailed boots, a very necessary form of footwear on the roads, the most important of which were very rough, laid with granite or elvan, which the roadmen, sitting all day behind their ever-growing piles of stones, cracked from huge blocks of rock with a small steel hammer mounted on a three-foot handle of ash plant. These cubes of broken stone, about two inches in every direction, were strewn from the tails of carts and levelled on the hard road surface by a shovel. Owing to the small number of steam rollers available, very few of these stones were ever pressed into place, and on newly-laid patches horses had to walk, keeping as close to the side of the road as possible.

I cannot imagine how the shoes of modern ladies, equipped with long spiked heels would fare on such roads.

Some of the farm women waiting on the doorstep would possibly have walked as much as nine or ten miles since daybreak and were faced with the same return journey, unless they were lucky enough to obtain a lift on a cart, or in a buggy.

The most depressing sound I can remember, one I used to hear so frequently between one and five o'clock in the morning, was the hoof beats of a horse trotting up our road as fast as its legs could carry it.

Outside our front gate the rider would jump off with a clatter of boots, drag his horse clop-clop up the cement path to the front door, hitch his reins over the post, then proceed to batter the door with his stick, while with his free hand he made a simultaneous assault on the chain which rang the night bell.

At the working end of this was a huge metal dome, which at one time had adorned the bridge of a ship. When it rang it disturbed not only my father, who was probably awake already, but also the neighbours for fifty yards around. The noise it made was so persistent and prolonged that when my father poked his head out of the bedroom window he would for some time be unable to hear a word the man was shouting.

Quite a lot of our clients were tin miners who worked underground by day and did their farming by night, or at least that part of it which their wives and daughters had been unable to deal with during the day. The following week or month, according to where they worked, they could farm by day and carry on underground by night.

When on day shift, they would return home at about five in the afternoon, work on the farm until ten or eleven in the winter months, and then by local custom they would habitually walk around their stock to make sure they were well and comfortable for the night.

Whether the eyesight of these miner-farmers was keener at that late hour, or whether darkness added to their fears is uncertain, but the fact remains that they could smell-out illness better at midnight than at any other time.

When once their fears were aroused it was considered the right thing, a matter of local etiquette presumably, to collect the neighbours, or as many as possible, even if it meant pulling them out of bed, to seek their advice. Almost invariably someone would suggest giving the poor beast, usually a cow, a pint of hot elder tea with two pounds of golden syrup stirred into it. After this had been poured down her throat, they would light their pipes and watch her for an hour to see what effect the mixture would produce.

At the end of this period it was customary to decide that this was "a case for the vet," and he, poor man, would be sent for.

By the time the messenger had caught a horse, especially when catching it meant patrolling a five acre field to find it, and after his wife had dressed and made him "a dish of tea" to keep out the cold, it would be well on to three o'clock in the morning before our ship's bell rang out the alarm.

If the veterinary surgeon had been lucky enough to get to bed that night, he would have to dress, saddle his horse, collect his kit for the saddlebags, probably tie some ropes and obstetric kit on his back, mount his horse and set out on his journey.

Most of us kept one or two horses in boxes close at hand, in readiness for night calls, their saddles and bridles laid out ready to put on.

Prior to the advent of the 'phone, which proved to be no unmixed blessing, we were called out three or four nights out of the seven, sometimes more than once during a night; or we would arrive home to find another horse hitched to the gatepost and another farm hand waiting with a message. What was worse was to hear the clatter of hoofs half-an-hour after one had got back into a warm bed!

Never on any night did the veterinary surgeon, or for that matter, the country doctor, close his eyes with that delightful certainty which would have induced relaxation and restful sleep. More often than not one lay half-asleep, ever listening, until the demand for sleep became overpowering.

With the coming of the 'phone, one could not claim to be pulled out of bed so frequently, for now it was so easy for the farmer to 'phone, one so seldom ever got into it. I used to think that the sudden explosive ringing of the telephone bell at the side of one's bed was more nerve-wracking than the clip clop of horses' feet trotting up the road. It was so difficult to forget the 'phone's presence in the darkness and to submerge the impression that scores of your clients might already be converging upon their own, like evil spirits determined to destroy your comfort and drag you forth into the freezing darkness.

Another change which occurred on the farm as the result of the introduction of the telephone, was that instead of it being etiquette to gather the neighbours and seek their advice, one got through to the veterinary surgeon right away and sought *his* advice, putting down the 'phone with the cheery remark, "Thanks, awfully. I'll see if she is any better in an hour's time and if she isn't, I'll ring again and ask you to come out."

Two or three such conversations shortly after climbing into bed did not act as a tranquiliser, and in the end it seemed easier to dress and settle down in an armchair until the summons came.

There is no comparison between the amount of nightwork fifty years ago and today, and it was so different having to saddle a horse and set out often into almost complete darkness, to what it is nowadays when one jumps into a car, turns on the headlights and the heater, and may be back in bed in a little over an hour. Moreover, night calls are becoming a thing of the past.

Outside the West country, few modern farmers trudge around their stock at night. The Cornish smallholder would have been very hard hit if he had lost a sixty pound cow through want of a little care. Nowadays, it doesn't matter so much, the farmer has struck more prosperous times.

During my third year in practice on my own account, I achieved a record in the eyes, at least, of my fellow practitioners, and the local doctors. Many tried to dig up a similar achievement but so far is I remember nobody quite scored over me. There is one thing certain, that if it was not surpassed in those days, the feat never will be again.

I take no pride in it, in fact most of the time I hated what I was doing. Briefly stated, I rode a relay of horses for twenty-one days and nights on urgent visits, with only one night, the tenth, in bed.

During this long spell, I arrived back at my surgery a number of times to collect more messages. I even got half-way up the stairs once or twice with the intention of tumbling into bed, but I was always thwarted.

In my area there were seventy cows calving on each day throughout the year on an average. Actually more did this in summer than in winter, so one might claim that eighty-five calved each summer day and night and fifty-five day and night during the winter. Apart from calving difficulties, parturition might be followed by milk fever, prolapse of the uterus, retained membranes, or symptoms of ketosis.

Milk fever was one of the diseases which demanded the most urgent attendance and this occurred most frequently in spring and early summer when the grass was growing rapidly. During my so very busy three weeks, the weather had been particularly moist and warm, the grass *was* green and growing, and cows went down with milk fever in every direction.

Fortunately for me, as well as for my clients, on the twenty-first day a cold east wind sprang up with some ground frost. The grass stopped growing, the cows ceased to develop hypocalcaemia—to give milk fever its correct name—and a very weary veterinary surgeon staggered into bed.

But with the passing of the years a change came over the means of transport and this change affected veterinary practice in a number of ways.

The horse, which had held sway from time immemorial, began to give place to the mechanised vehicle. The number of horses in the country began gradually to decrease and country veterinary practice entered a new era.

There were people, even in those days, who took a dismal view of the future. The boldest among them prophesied that in years to come the horse would give way on the roads to the motor-propelled vehicle.

This suggestion split the country into two camps: those who could not imagine the town and countryside without its horses, and those who maintained that although horses would always be cheaper to maintain, motor vehicles would come into universal favour. A great many saw that money was to be made out of motor cars and they set into motion propaganda against the slow, obsolete horse.

But even veterinary surgeons, who should have fought tooth

and nail to save it, were among the first to discard the horse in favour of the more speedy vehicle. No longer were we all content to ride or drive their forty miles a day and visit an average of eight farms in the twenty four hours. Some of us acquired motor cycles, most dangerous contraptions, fitted with fixed gears and a high frame, brakes of doubtful efficiency, and control cables which went out of action at critical moments.

I remember, with my first machine, how I used to run beside it to start the engine, then with a flying leap one travelled horizontally through the air clinging madly to the handlebars, and if lucky eventually landed astride the saddle.

If one were better favoured one acquired in place of the motor cycle a single cylinder car of six to eight horse power, often depending for its vitality upon a relay of accumulators. As the lighting was by paraffin or carbide, the batteries were required only for ignition, but to tell the truth, they lasted the single cylinder engine much longer than one would imagine.

Of course, the car was by no means as fast as the motor cycle but think of the comfort, the luxury of a leather covered bucket seat, a canvas hood which could be pulled up when it rained, and a glass windscreen to keep off the wind.

Those among us who were determined to keep up with the times, and hang the expense, used to chug chug along the roads, with much crashing of gears, at a speed often approaching thirty miles an hour; on a good level road it must be understood.

We began to travel greater distances from the surgery and this introduced a spirit of competition between local practitioners, both medical and veterinary. It was not long before two of either profession, formerly the best of friends, would begin to cut each other dead as they met on their rounds.

This extension of practice boundaries at first was not attended by the happiest of relationships, but in time as motor vehicles became more dependable and faster, it gradually became recognised that practices no longer possessed boundaries as of yore, and that instead of one practitioner possessing a local monopoly, clients were in a position to choose their professional man, doctor, or veterinary surgeon, and were no longer obliged to employ the nearest.

In course of time most of us became the proud possessors of "Tin Lizzies," and for ever after we owed a debt of gratitude to Henry Ford.

It took only a few years for the country doctor and the country veterinary surgeon to become completely car-minded. The horse, growing older, was turned out to graze, as the new chauffeur felt that horseflesh was beneath his notice. It was brought in and given a feed of corn only when hounds were due to meet in the vicinity, for in spite of this new-found love for the motor car, the vehicle could not carry one across country and the horse needed some exercise, anyway.

Very soon, however, professional men acquired the jargon of the seasoned motorist, and they competed with each other in acquring the latest models and were as conceited about these as they had ever been about their horses.

When previously, meeting over a drink or a game of cards, doctor and veterinary surgeon had "talked horses," they now no longer spoke of these discarded animals. They talked about their motor cars and congratulated themselves, forty years ago, on having been born at a time which enabled them during their lives to enjoy all the pleasures attainable in the age of motor car perfection.

In these days a fillip was given to country practice because professional people could get through their work so much faster, leaving more time for rest and recreation, hobbies and the social pleasures hitherto denied them.

Both the country doctor and the country veterinary surgeon were the proud possessors of a few alarming and insanitary instruments, a collection of drugs not necessarily lethal if used with due discrimination, probably less dangerous than many in common use today.

There were few hospitals, possibly a cottage hospital serving a considerable area, and no fit accommodation for surgical cases. Doctors operated on the kitchen table or in some cases while the patient lay in his bed.

But neither doctor nor veterinary surgeon could have been accused of ignorance for at that period there was very little, apart from anatomy, that one could know. Research lay in the future and bothered nobody, while a great deal that was universally accepted as fact was based on heresy and superstition. Undoubtedly the graduates of future generations will pass exactly the same criticism regarding the graduates of this present one.

But neither of these professional men was at all conscious of his shortcomings. Each possessed a colossal belief in himself and his own importance. He had descended from his horse; the influence of motordom was making itself felt.

But although the old-time practitioners, human and animal doctors, were far behind those of the present day in scientific knowledge, each had a very good idea whether the patient was likely to live or die, with or in spite of treatment. Such knowledge was not a matter of intuition but it was based, even if subconsciously, on experience rather than upon accurate diagnosis or scientific reasoning.

The days of organised and extensive enquiry into human and animal disease, of intensive research and experimental surgery, were yet to come.

In the outlying districts of Cornwall even witchcraft flourished, and in my boyhood days I had first-hand evidence of the way the witches worked and the results they achieved.

In the south-west the witches enjoyed the advantages of local superstition. So many illnesses, of which we now know the causation and can apply the appropriate treatment, were ascribed to the influence of the evil eye. The animals or the people had been "overlooked," and it was a matter of common agreement among country folk that such disorders were not of the kind which doctors or veterinary surgeons could deal with; they were essentially the business of the witches, to be treated by charms, or some form of black magic.

When there were two witches in the district, as there were in one particular area within my practice, the one witch would be employed to lay on the curses, and the other to lift them off, all for a suitable consideration.

I had a strong suspicion that in spite of the antipathy expressed by the one for the other, and vice versa at every public opportunity, these two ladies had probably entered into a secret partnership and were reaping a communal harvest.

Cows were alleged to be suffering either from "bladder under the tongue," or from "worm in the tail," according to choice, or perhaps according to which end of the animal appeared to carry the greater burden of illness. In either case the cure was the same.

The tongue would be raised and the fraenum sliced with a knife and blood would be drawn, or the tail would be lifted and a razor drawn across the subcaudal artery. In each case salt would be rubbed freely into the wounds.

It would be reckoned a sheer waste of time to call in the veterinary surgeon when the cause was so obvious and the remedy so simple. If after all this the animal died, one had no cause for reproach. Everything possible had been done.

The witches were not occupied solely with veterinary patients. They could charm warts off the farmer's hands, stop his nose from bleeding, or cure the wife's housemaid's knee. They had no particular need even to see the patient.

For those who could be circumspect and were willing to pay well for the service, far greater miracles could be arranged for.

One's personal enemies could be removed from the world, never to return even in spirit shape. If it were preferable, an enemy could be ruined and brought to starvation by the use of charms which would destroy his cattle or his poultry, or even his relations. To effect this worthy purpose, it was necessary only for the client to obtain by some means a small quantity of the potential victim's urine, or other excrement. This was mixed with clay into a rough effigy of the person, or even of the animal, it was proposed should be punished, or liquidated.

A needle inserted at suitable depth into an appropriate part of the clay body, would produce specific results and guarantee an injury. Sticking the needle into the region of the heart of the model would ensure sudden death of the original.

However, before we scoff at these charlatans of past days we must remember that at the present time educated people, otherwise apparently sane, place equal reliance on mystical "boxes" containing no batteries or "works" of any kind, plentifully besprinkled with dummy switches; machines, which when presented with a hair or a drop of saliva, or blood from a horse or dog, will, after the turning of a few knobs, present one with a report which will describe the disease from which the animal is presumed to suffer and its appropriate treatment. These machines are probably a great deal less efficacious than the arts of the witches. The latter could at least exert some psychological influence which sometimes produced miracles in its own peculiar fashion.

The surgery of fifty years ago, both human and animal, was perhaps a little crude by modern standards, but it was based on fairly sound concepts. Although surgical sites were frequently swamped with strong disinfectants, the old-time surgeons were firm believers in the efficient drainage of their wounds so it is likely that potentially harmful disinfectants escaped with the discharges.

Physiology capered with superstition and bio-chemistry, as we now regard it, was in its infancy. There were, however, some veterinary physiologists ahead of their times, and foremost among these one may pick out General Sir Fred Smith, who although he concentrated largely on horses, the animals he knew so well, wrote a book on veterinary physiology which makes good reading today.

One must make due allowance for the fact that the veterinary surgeon of half-a-century ago possessed a number of natural advantages denied to the present generation, particularly as regards his upbringing prior to his college training.

The present day university student may attain his Tripos and then be called upon to decide which profession, out of a number, he will choose for further study.

He may select the veterinary calling for a variety of reasons, the two foremost being that it is not (yet) nationalised, and because those who practise it nowadays usually earn large incomes. There is no reference here, you will notice, to any special ability or any background suggesting special affection for animals, or any prior knowledge of them, of their habits, characteristics, or mentality.

When these young men eventually graduate they will undoubtedly turn out to be good scientists and will approach all their professional problems in an intelligent and scientific manner. But during their first ten years in practice they will labour in one sense under an inferiority complex, because they will be employed by animal owners who will lack scientific knowledge in most cases, but will be thoroughly at home with animals and how to approach them, handle them and humour them. I have heard quite a number of young veterinary surgeons in practice confess that they were "scared stiff of horses," and greatly disliked having to attend them.

This is entirely due to the fact that they have never during their young days had any contact with horses and perhaps with no other animals either, and it is a fact that unless children associate with animals from infancy onwards they seldom feel quite at home in their company.

How this can be overcome is a problem which gives food for thought. It is perfectly true that young veterinary graduates who are called in to hunting, stud and racing stables to attend horses, lack the ability of the stable lads in handling them, however much they may have learned about their diseases.

In the universities students have little contact with horses, and university teachers are seldom practical horsemen, however much they may shine as teachers.

The lad of 1900 often rode his pony several miles to school, was born a horseman among horsemen, and living in a country village or on a farm, had become accustomed to farm animals and dogs from the day he could toddle. This kind of education can be provided no longer except in very exceptional cases.

The modern youth passes from prep. school, into a public school and then into a university. His vacations will be spent with his parents, possibly abroad on holiday, and unless his father, and perhaps his mother, take an interest in hunting or racing, it is unlikely they, or he, will have any animal interests.

It becomes necessary, therefore, for the new graduate when confronted by an animal patient, to regard it as though it were a creature almost strange to him. He must decide upon its breed, its sex and, of course, its species, on sight. He has then to conjure up in his mind the structure of this particular animal by recollection of his anatomical studies, now some years behind him.

He will probably keep his distance from it, and view it from afar, because he is a little uncertain of the temperament common to the species when encountered in the world outside the university walls, and very wisely, perhaps, prefers to let someone else approach it before he exposes himself to undue risk.

It would be quite unfair to belittle the modern graduate because he is less familiar than his predecessors with the animals he is called upon to treat. It would be quite wrong, too, to persist nowadays in the old adage that "horsemen are born, not made." It never *was* true, and is less so today than ever. The present day graduate has had little opportunity to learn something which the older people acquired quite unconsciously.

Most university schools now run field stations where students see a small selection of animals; they seldom make sufficiently close contact with them to become familiar with handling them, and there may be nobody at the field station to provide instruction in the art. It is true that animal husbandry is taught, and in the old days this was catered for by a subject that was referred to as "Animal Management." The examination fifty years ago in this subject was very practical. Candidates had to saddle horses, harness them, even in pairs, remove shoes, spot lameness, and be able to age and describe any animal presented. The examiners were veterinary surgeons who were well-known as practical horsemen. Failure in this branch of the examination even in those days held up quite a number of students who had been reared in towns. I remember one student who had failed this examination on three occasions, putting him back eighteen months. He was then provided with a special tutor. On the fourth attempt, he gained full marks for horsemanship, harnessing and mounting and dismounting. Unfortunately his marks were finally reduced to nil, because he had worked always from the right side (then the "off" side) of the horse instead of the left (the near side).

Veterinary students spend some part of their vacations in practice with veterinary surgeons, but this does not always provide the amount of experience it should do. Few principals have the time, and not always the inclination, to act as extra-mural teachers, and students are often handed over to young assistants who cannot teach them a great deal.

The medical student possesses considerable advantages in this respect as he has the hospital wards, and only one animal to deal with; one, too, with which he has become familiar since birth.

There is no doubt that a year spent working in stables and on a farm before going to university, is one answer to many of these problems, but as the university course is a long one the extra time spent in this way is not always consistent with economics, particularly when a father has several children to launch into the world.

In our earlier days the horse was the universal plaything as well as the essential means of transport and conveyer of draught. In those days, too, whether the country lad became a doctor, a veterinary surgeon, a parson or a bank clerk, he remained always a horseman. Quite often, so far as his circumstances permitted, he continued to ride and even breed horses, watch them and study them from every angle.

His attention had not then been diverted by space travel, not even by transatlantic flight and certainly not by jet propulsion, or the disintegration of the atom, which if it were ever discussed at all, was dismissed as a myth of the first magnitude.

Not only the veterinary surgeon but his friends, whether or not they were also his clients, were all equally at home with horses, dogs and probably with farm animals also. Unless the ability to size up the animal, handle it, observe features of conformation and the signs of disease, was better developed in the veterinary surgeon than in the client, he soon ceased to function as adviser to the latter.

The human patient can talk and answer questions, tell the doctor where he, or she, feels the pain, which limb hurts most, and provide other information.

When the country doctor of fifty years ago visited a patient on the farm he might bleed him, stick a few leeches on certain parts of the body to keep him awake, then rattle him back to the cottage hospital in an iron-tyred buggy over atrocious roads.

Today he dispatches him to a large central hospital in an oxygen chamber fitted inside an ambulance which is well sprung on pneumatic tyres; perhaps he is given a blood transfusion enroute. By the time the patient arrives he will be fortified by the injection of one or two antibiotics with some hydrocortisone and the latest tranquilizer.

In spite of all this the patient often survives; the human being is an adaptable animal. The variation in treatment as compared with that of former years, spells progress.

The veterinary profession is not one whit behind its sister profession in the matter of knowledge and scientific research into animal disease, and this is specially manifested in the great advances made in small animal practice discussed at the International Conference, sponsored by the British Small Animal Veterinary Congress, and held in London during April 1961.

The discussions were held at a very high level and were participated in by delegates from the United Kingdom, the United States of America and most of the Continental countries. A perusal of the journal *Advances in Small Animal Practice* Volume III, which gives full particulars of the papers contributed, will provide better evidence of the position which veterinary science has now attained than can be proffered in any other way.

The only factor which limits the amount of professional attention which can be afforded to animal patients is that of cost. Human life is supposed to be of sufficient value to justify remedial measures regardless of expense, but animal treatment is always a matter of how much the owner is willing or capable to spend on treatment. This implies no desire on the part of the veterinary surgeon to charge more than he can help doing, but as dogs require the same dose of a medicine or antibiotic as a man, the application of modern treatments is apt to be expensive. However, very few owners of animals ever consider the cost when the life of a pet is at stake.

In the case of other animals on the farm, the matter of economics plays a greater part. The veterinary profession is becoming more and more specialised and when animals are particularly valuable, or sentiment makes them so, the services of specialists in various disorders can be engaged.

The young graduate may become a clinician, a teacher or a research worker. He may become attached to a pharmaceutical firm and devote his studies to the development of newer or better drugs, he may enter a laboratory or occupy a post under the Ministry of Agriculture, acting as a whole or part-time inspector attached to the Animal Health Division.

The majority of new graduates enroll as assistants, eventually become partners and spend their whole lives in general practice, acting also in most instances as part time local veterinary inspectors to the same Ministry.

Apart from these outlets, if he, or she, wishes to specialise in any branch of medicine or surgery, or in pathology, bacteriology, or any of the sciences, in such items as kidney diseases, pediatrics or genetics, there is usually scope for such a departure in one of the large composite practices, of which every member specialises in one subject, in addition to acting as a participant in general practice. Most large practices now carry up-to-date laboratories, where bacteriology, haemotology, urine examination, the diagnosis of skin diseases and of parasitic diseases, are dealt with as a part of the practice routine.

It is unfortunate that workers who specialise purely in research are still too badly paid, in all the professions, to make the project as attractive as it should be. There are a great many young graduates who have dedicated themselves to carrying out certain lines of research who, financially, are worse off than the well-paid graduate who takes an assistantship in a veterinary practice.

Chapter Three

SETTING UP IN PRACTICE

I<small>T IS PRESUMED</small> that the young veterinary surgeon imbued with the commendable intention of setting up in practice on his own account, entertains no illusions concerning what lies ahead of him, even in these days of luxurious living. It is to be hoped he does not anticipate a life of undiluted pleasure and is not averse to a little chastisement of the flesh.

So many practitioners discover as they journey through life that the demands made upon them by clients and circumstances are far heavier than they had anticipated. They may then find themselves gyrating in the whirlpool of veterinary practice with the rapids constantly drawing nearer. Many are so busily engaged in their daily toil that they are carried away before they have time to take heed, sometimes in the literal sense, sometimes in the metaphorical.

All people have not the gift of martyrdom, and although it is true that a genuine liking for one's task helps to ease the burden of unceasing labour, it is undoubtedly a fact that veterinary practice can become very wearisome to those who enter into it with the sole object of earning a living. Unless a young graduate is content to devote his whole life and leisure ungrudgingly to the care and treatment of animals regardless of self, he will be well advised to direct his energies towards some branch other than active practice.

Fortunately, there are often other posts open to him. One of these is to remain at his university and devote his time to teaching. In this case he will be wise never to make the break from within the university walls even to see some practice, since a short absence may cause him to be forgotten while another graduate steps into his place.

The main advantage he would gain by spending at least a short time in general practice would be to gain some idea of the amount of hard work in entails. Having once worked in this way he might thereafter be more content to cope with the boredom which comes from routine tasks, with a lot of time to waste, either in the university, or within the walls of a building devoted to the sale of pharmaceutical products. He would discover also that the practical man who earns his experience the hard way is less honoured by his professional brethren than he who is brimful of academic knowledge gained by much reading.

As a salaried worker in some sphere other than practice, he would enjoy regular hours, holidays without fears, he would retire on a pension while still an active man, even if afterwards he were compelled to vegetate woefully and exist in straitened circumstances until death released him.

I have always advised every young man before entering the veterinary profession with the intention of sitting up in general practice to undergo a stringent medical examination to determine if he is sufficiently well-endowed both physically and mentally to undertake a life task which demands strenous and exhausting labour, long hours and the expenditure of much nervous energy. He must be fit to turn out of a warm bed, drive many miles, strip to the skin on the coldest night, work to the point of complete exhaustion, drive home, sleep, and be up and ready for more early the same morning.

Temperaments vary greatly, and it is quite evident to one who had enjoyed a long experience of veterinary practice and veterinary surgeons, that the endocrine system and the mental equilibrium of every young man is not calculated to withstand the stresses inseparable from veterinary practice in the cowshed and the field.

While the introverts among us become neurotic, develop duodenal ulcers and hypertension, and end up as perambulating invalids at forty, the extroverts appear to be immune to worry. Trouble bounces off them leaving no visible scars. Unfortunately, as with mushrooms and marriage, by the time one discovers one has made a mistake, it is too late.

The right time to consult a doctor and a psychiatrist is before the irrevocable step is taken.

I have a feeling, too, that in the veterinary world, as in some other equally respected callings, celibacy should be encouraged.

This is not because I do not value the help a good wife can give, but because being a confirmed feminist, with the greatest admiration for the wives of veterinary surgeons whom I have met, I am certain they are getting a raw deal.

The majority of these ladies not only listened to their husbands' grumbling and shared their burdens, but they also ran the homes, looked after the waiting room, consulting room and pharmacy, answered continuous 'phone calls, pacified querulous clients, and kept the books in their spare time. All of them may not undertake *all* these tasks, but even so, I feel sure in my heart that it is neither right nor kind for a young veterinary surgeon contemplating general practice to ask any woman's hand in marriage.

Do not imagine, however, that any of these drawbacks will deter the lady of your choice if you do happen to ask.

The majority of young veterinary surgeons commence as assistants, find a practice they like, enter into partnership and eventually succeed to the practice on the retirement or death of the principal.

On the other hand the graduate may purchase an existing practice, one from which the present owner wishes to retire through age, or illness. Purchase in such circumstances is not without risk since the clients may have migrated to neighbouring practitioners, and also because the new graduate may find it a little difficult to follow in the footsteps of a more experienced practitioner.

Veterinary practice has several facets and the doctoring of sick animals is only one of them.

A capacity for organisation and business management, an appreciation of the science of economics, unbounded energy plus a love of order, tidiness and cleanliness of place and person, all are required if the newcomer is to carry on successfully and dodge bankruptcy.

It is equally as important to be what is known as a "good mixer," as it is for the doctor to cultivate the correct "bedside manner." The tactful handling of clients will keep many a practitioner solvent even if his professional skill does not attain the same level.

The other way of commencing a practice—not one greatly

favoured in high places—is to find a suitable locality where veterinary surgeons are scarce—not easy, nowadays—put up one's plate, and wait.

The man who does this must realize that his coming must be silent and unaccompanied by a flourish of trumpets. The ethical code of the Royal College of Veterinary Surgeons does not permit the newcomer to advertise his presence, either in the local newspaper, or by any other means. His plate must be small, and as insignificant as possible.

At the same time he must do all he can to meet and establish friendly relationship with neighbouring veterinary surgeons, and persuade them, if possible, to secure him nomination for membership of the local division of the British Veterinary Association. He must sink or swim according to the reputation he acquires as the result of his attendance upon the animals which may be brought to him, but he must also remain very awake to the fact that clients dissatisfied with their previous veterinary surgeons, as well as those not actively dissatisfied but a little curious concerning "the new veterinary surgeon," may bring pets for his treatment which are at the time the patients of some other veterinary surgeon. This is a trap which our young man will have to avoid.

Few lay persons have any conception of the severity with which the ethical code of the profession may be enforced.

It is often difficult to make a worried owner understand that he, or she, being already the client of another veterinary surgeon, cannot take a sick animal elsewhere when it is already receiving professional treatment, unless he or she pays the account of the veterinary surgeon already in attendance and intimates that his services are no longer required. In such circumstances the newcomer should insist on seeing the animal in consultation with the veterinary surgeon previously in attendance, and make no attempt to deprive him of his client.

To criticise the treatment or the behaviour of another veterinary surgeon is considered conduct disgraceful in the professional sense and it is likely to bring down severe penalties upon the transgressor.

Defaulting veterinary surgeons may be brought before the Disciplinary Committee of the Royal College of Veterinary Surgeons who may erase their names from the Register.

Clients, distressed at the thought of possibly losing their pets, cast aside all scruples, and the veterinary surgeon, unless he has the gift of second sight, may be deceived. The veterinary surgeon must be very careful that sentiment or sympathy do not permit him to accept patients without a deal of tactful questioning.

When I started practice in my twenty-second year by "putting up my plate" in a terrace of a small Cornish town, I had the advantage that I was only about ten miles from the town in which my father was practising, and I was able to call him in consultation whenever I came up against a case with which, owing to lack of experience, I was unable to cope. This gave both my client and myself confidence.

Any success I attained in building up a practice of considerable size was due partly to the fact that veterinary surgeons were scarce in the area, but in no small measure it was due to the help afforded me by my father, quite as much as to my own efforts.

Until this time most of the local farmers had depended upon quacks and intinerant medicine vendors. I have nothing to say against the former, or at least the majority of them. They were experienced men and even if their scientific knowledge was small, and though their treatments were simple and often savoured of magic, they seldom did much harm. It cannot be denied that these men knew a great deal about animals, irrespective of their ailments.

There were specialists among them, too; the castrators of horses and bulls, the castrators of pigs and the spayers, and there were those who calved cows and lambed ewes. The same men seldom undertook more than the one kind of task.

Some of the older men among them were remarkably good obstetricians. They were very particular about their ropes, their few instruments and their blocks and pulleys. They were skillful and gentle in their manipulations; they used pounds of pure lard and gallons of boiled linseed as lubricants. The mortality rate among their patients was surprisingly low.

Although I did not always welcome their ministrations, I admired their skill. These men had never heard of a Caesarian operation before I performed some from 1917 onwards, and I had to agree with them, and still do, that an experienced obstetrician can safely calve 95 per cent of all dystocia cases quite successfully by internal manipulation and controlled traction. The present day embryotomes make the operation even easier. I averaged about seven difficult calvings each week and the number of Caesarians were seldom more than two or three in a year.

At the time I first put up my plate the surrounding country was very wild and undeveloped in the true farming sense, but it carried natural pasture and it was estimated that my own area contained 25,000 dairy cattle, not counting beef cattle, together with 3,500 horses, not including the ponies running wild on the moors, and the hundreds of half-starved animals employed in carting tin ore at the mines.

As the practice grew I took a partner, and we kept several qualified assistants, as well as a number of lay helpers in the surgery and yard, office and dispensary.

The practice I left nearly twenty years ago before moving north, continues to flourish under management better than it received during my own tenancy. But conditions have changed. The radio car has removed the farm women from the doorstep and in place of the farmers' wives turning up in their hobnailed boots they now drive up in new modern cars, and in getting out to enter the surgery display a length of nylon stocking and stiletto-heeled shoes, another clear indication of progress.

The surrounding country has changed also, and I doubt if the younger members of the firm can imagine the conditions which existed when twenty tin mines were in full work in the neighbourhood, long before motor cars came into general use.

The population has increased greatly since mining came almost to a standstill, and the townspeople and villagers concentrated on attracting visitors to the beautiful Cornish coast. With the rise in population the local demand for dairy produce, poultry, meat and fish has increased also, now there are more mouths to be fed, all of which necessitates additional veterinary service.

But I can claim at least that I was the pioneer.

It was my role early in my professional career to educate the local farmers and horseowners into a proper appreciation of the value of veterinary service. This was equivalent to making them understand that a guinea spent, often meant sixty saved. This does not imply that on occasion both the one and the sixty did not roll down the drain in company.

These were the occasions when the tactful handling of clients came to the rescue and prevented loss of faith. Farmers and horse-owners may have their sentimental moments but these are not particularly evident when they find themselves losing money. Before I had been in practice a year I was fully convinced that the clients must see a good return for their expenditure, or else it was the knacker or the butcher who would reap the reward which should have come to the veterinary surgeon.

Young practitioners, when first they make contact with their clients, may be lucky or unlucky, in spite of their efforts and intentions. Quite frequently neither skill nor foresight has anything to do with the kind of impression they make in the eyes of their clients. I remember always one of my own early experiences, one which has helped to convince me ever since, that it is better to be born lucky than rich.

My plate had been up only a few weeks when a farmer from a village, nine miles distant, asked me to call and examine a sick cow. He said she seemed unable to raise her head from the ground.

When first I saw the animal, the owner's description seemed very appropriate. She was evidently in great distress and her nose seemed as though glued to the ground. Her breathing was painful and each expiration was accompanied by a loud grunt. Saliva dribbled constantly from the corners of her mouth.

When I had spent all the time I dared to do in making my examination, striving desperately to arrive at a diagnosis, the farmer remarked that now "after all that," he would like to know what ailed his cow.

I was in exactly the same state of mind as he was, but unfortunately it was now my turn to speak.

A little rashly, perhaps, I told him I suspected she had swallowed a foreign body. This conveyed little to his imagination and he demanded to know what was a foreign body?

I explained that this was a scientific term which might include such objects as a nail, a piece of iron wire, a screw, and/or a screwdriver. I was running a little short of foreign bodies by this time but hurriedly I thought of another—a sheet of tin!

I fear my client was not greatly impressed and after I had explained to him that nothing in my stock of drugs was likely to make any impression on a fragment of ironmongery hidden in the cow's interior, I departed for home, a little saddened. I told myself it was unlikely I would ever visit this farm again.

But I was wrong in thinking in this way. A fortnight later I received a telegram from my client. It read:

"Come immediately to open up cow."

This shook me a little. I was only too sadly aware that in proffering my diagnosis I was drawing a bow at a venture, and never for one moment had I dreamed I might be called up to substantiate my opinion.

I got on my horse and proceeded to the farm. When I was within a mile of it I was surprised at the local activity. Horses and traps seemed to be everywhere; a few farmers were pedalling along on bicycles with much bell-ringing, all heading in the same direction as myself.

It shook me a great deal more when I came into sight of the farmyard and saw that it was filled and overflowing with folk. I imagined I must have made some mistake and wandered into a farm auction.

But no! The gathering was arranged in my honour and all these people had collected at the farm to see the "foreign body" which the "new vet." was about to extract from the remains of Farmer Richard's best cow.

The carcase lay in state on a pile of manure in the centre of the farmyard. Grouped all around it were men munching pasties and passing around large pitchers of cider from which everyone drank in turn. An Irish wake had nothing on this ceremony. Nobody passed me a pitcher.

By the side of the body of the deceased cow stood the knacker, an unpleasant looking man of gross fatness, adorned with a beard. In his right hand he brandished a huge knife, mounted in a bone handle, and between his teeth he gripped the steel, upon which at intervals he proposed apparently to whet its blade.

I could see when his gaze first alighted upon my countenance that he was the kind of man who held veterinary surgeons in no great esteem, in fact he appeared markedly antagonistic. When I surveyed him standing there with that knife in his hand I experienced a chilly sensation running downwards, the length of my spine.

Without even a "good morning" he proceeded to "open up" the cow.

He sliced through the hide along the whole length of the abdomen, and pushed his huge hand beneath it.

"Nothing there!" he bellowed, in a voice that could have been heard all over the parish.

He divided the abdominal muscles throughout their length.

"Nothing there!" he cried.

He cut through the abdominal tunic, severing the peritoneum in one swipe of the knife, and dived his arm into the peritoneal cavity. "Nothing there!" He repeated his stock phrase a number of times while he dragged the stomachs into view, slashed them open and dived his hand into the various parts.

"Nothing anywhere!" he bawled, with an air of finality.

I cast a quick searching glance around that crowding sea of faces, and I didn't care a great deal for the expressions I saw on some of them.

These men had sacrificed half-a-day's work, almost bringing the local mine to a stand still, and what was there to show for it?

"Nothing anywhere!" the knacker shouted again as though he read their thoughts.

Only the knacker was looking really pleased. I could see very clearly it was my turn to do something—and quickly!

In desperation I took up the knife the knacker had laid beside the carcase and cut through the diaphragm, laying open the chest cavity. And I knew I was saved! I had felt the grate of metal on metal.

With the finest air of nonchalance I could muster, I introduced my hand into the chest and like a conjuror producing a rabbit, I drew out a piece of galvanised iron four inches in length, shaped like a miniature sickle. Running through the rim and protruding an inch from either end was a stout iron wire. This was evidently a portion of the rim of a pail, one which had been discarded and had almost rusted away.

How the cow managed to swallow anything of this size and shape is difficult to understand. The fact that she did so has endeared her within my memory ever since.

What I am certain about is that the presence of that slice of pail exactly where I wanted it, made the accuracy of my diagnosis the chief topic of conversation for miles around, and from then on my professional standing was assured.

Nowadays, of course, I could have verified my diagnosis from the commencement by the use of an instrument based on the army mine detector. I could have operated on the cow in the early stages and possibly have saved her life. But I didn't.

I doubt, however, if the most successful operation would have enhanced my reputation to the same degree as the result of that post-mortem succeeded in doing.

One of the things every doctor and veterinary surgeon has to avoid is that which might possibly be regarded as advertising. In this particular instance I think I could hardly have been found guilty.

Chapter Four

SOME DISEASES OF ANIMALS

Now that I have told you how busy we were always kept, I would like to mention a few of the illnesses of cattle which took up a great deal of our time.

I will discuss parturition difficulties in a later chapter, but the few diseases I will briefly mention counted among the commoner kinds of trouble.

One of the illnesses which occurred extremely freely among the high-yielding Guernsey cows, particularly these with a particularly high butter fat milk content was the condition known as milk fever, which arises from a deficiency of calcium in the blood stream. Normally, the long bones serve as reservoirs of calcium and the mineral can be transferred to the blood as required, the regulating mechanism lying in the parathyroid gland. If anything goes wrong with the functioning of this gland the transfer of calcium from bone to blood may not take place sufficiently rapidly. The muscles become rigid, the cow totters about and soon falls to the ground, becomes comatose and may die fairly quickly unless extra calcium is pumped by artificial means into the blood stream.

This disease was the bugbear of the Cornish farmers and in my boyhood days before the calcium theory was recognised cows were treated with neat whiskey and doses of chloral hydrate, mixed with golden syrup or treacle.

In my donkey-riding days my father would frequently be called in to a number of these cases every day, particularly during spring and summer and, of course, they provided a great deal of night work. When I mention that a case due to recover usually stayed on the ground about nine or more days and needed veterinary attendance daily, it becomes apparent that the veterinary surgeons were kept on the run. The mortality rate under the whiskey treatment was very high, as much as 75 per cent of cattle affected, but as a bottle of whiskey cost three and sixpence, a lot of money in those days, it was quite a popular method of treatment among the farm hands.

Two or three had to stay on duty by day and by night in order to keep the cow propped up on her brisket, with sacks filled with straw pushed between her shoulders and the ground. The head was also fastened to a beam by means of a rope tied around the cow's horns. If the cow succeeded in getting flat on her side as she constantly tried to do, her stomach would become distended with gas and she would die of suffocation.

Milk fever was responsible for the financial ruin of a good many farmers and there was universal rejoicing among them when Schmidt, in about 1900, discovered that cows recovered if about half-a-pint of lukewarm water in which a small quantity of iodide of potassium had been dissolved, was injected into each quarter of the udder via the teat canal. This fluid was left in the udder for 24 hours when it was milked out. The cow frequently recovered and was on her feet by the time she was due to be milked.

It was not long before veterinary surgeons found that the iodide of potassium played no useful part, and plain warm water was equally efficient. The recovery was due to pressure within the udder limiting or suppressing milk secretion with the result that calcium salts were not drained away from the body into the milk.

Following this discovery it was found that when the udder was inflated tightly with air and the teats tied with tape to prevent leakage, the cow would usually be up and well after an interval of only about four hours in most cases.

This treatment was a godsend to the farmer who ceased to lose one or two of his best cows each year.

Then Drs. Dryerre and Greig, two Scottish veterinary surgeons, demonstrated that milk fever was caused by a fall in the ratio of blood calcium and that very rapid recovery followed the injection of a soluble calcium salt into the blood stream. Calcium chloride was first used but proved to be too irritating to the vein and tissues. Is was succeeded by calcium borogluconate which has been employed successfully ever since.

When the calcium borogluconate treatment first came into vogue, we spent hours every day and often far into the night, boiling and filtering calcium into sterilised bottles. Soon, however, the drug firms saw a chance of doing business and they commenced to sell the solution in sterile bottles ready for injection. When it was found by veterinary surgeons that a lack of blood phosphorus played a part in producing milk fever they added phosphates to the injection and also dextrose which combats ketosis. Today, we buy our calcium injection in soft, plastic containers we can hang up over the cow and allow the fluid to drip into her veins through a rubber tube attached to an intravenous needle.

Although the cause and remedy are so well-known, no efficient method of prevention has yet been discovered, and, so, milk fever continues to keep both veterinary surgeons and pharmaceutical firms busily employed.

Just as lack of blood calcium causes muscle tetany, followed by unconsciousness, a deficiency of magnesium in the blood gives rise to hysterical symptoms with epileptiform convulsions, often attended by almost instantaneous death in many instances. This, too, now we know its cause, can be controlled to some extent by the injection of magnesium salts, such as Epsom salts beneath the skin or, well diluted, it can be injected into a vein, but with great care as to rapid administration may set up heart fibrillation with resulting death.

Hypomagnesaemia, better known as "grass staggers" is in some districts a terrible scourge causing serious losses before there is time to treat all the patients.

I have dwelt a little on these two conditions because I doubt if our younger practitioners have any conception of the terrible losses of stock and capital which resulted before the cause and appropriate treatments became known. Nor can they imagine the strain upon the veterinary surgeons, surrounded by cases of milk fever and grass staggers, with no efficient remedy. Prior to the early years of the twentieth century farmers lost their most valuable cows with consistent regularity with the result that dairy farmers became so improverished they seldom made any attempt to pay the veterinary surgeons for prolonged efforts on their behalf.

As a result veterinary practice reached a low ebb, not in the matter of activity, but economically.

It is likely that the discovery of udder injection by Schmidt, followed by the inflation treatment, and later by calcium therapy as a result of the researches carried out by Dryerre and Greig, saved the dairy industry from complete breakdown. Without veterinary discoveries in this particular direction the "Drink More Milk" campaign would never have come into being.

When udder injection for the treatment of milk fever was first practiced, I lost one of my most valuable clients in an extraordinary manner.

His best cow went down with the disease and, as usual, he was very downhearted as he fully expected she would die after a protracted illness.

It was a day in February when the evenings became dark quite early. My client built a large tent around the cow which was lying in the middle of a field on the top of a hill about a hundred and fifty yards from his dwelling house.

When evening came on he decided to adjourn to the local inn for refreshment and consolation, leaving an old farm hand in charge of the cow.

It was just after his departure that I arrived on the scene and administered the new treatment, and to keep the cow warm, I covered her with a large white mackintosh sheet. At 9 p.m. the cow was looking much better and the farm hand decided he could safely reach the public house at the other end of the village, which would not be in view of his employer, have a quick pint of beer and be back again before his return.

But as it happened my client was worried about his cow, and he returned to the farm to take another look at her before closing time.

Apparently the "new treatment" had worked wonders with the cow.

When her owner had almost climbed the steep hill which led to the field in which he had left her lying, he beheld what he took to be an apparition, clad in white, approaching him, and in terror he turned round and bolted for home as fast as he could run. He was a stout man and it is unlikely he had run for years.

The cow, for such it was, still wrapped in the white sheet, must have been craving for company, for when she saw her master running away she decided to run faster and join him.

My poor client, hearing the footsteps coming ever closer, put on speed, reached his front door and collapsed on the doorstep. He was found an hour later in a comatose condition and was taken inside and put to bed. The doctor was hurriedly fetched but in spite of all treatment the patient died during the night without regaining consciousness.

Two of the diseases which have taken their toll of cattle in a big way for countless years are tuberculosis and Johne's disease.

In Cornwall, in which county I practised, both of these were very prevalent, in fact even outside this county the scourge of tubercle in cattle was reckoned as affecting one cow in every three.

Johne's disease, a wasting condition associated with intermittent or persistent diarrhoea, probably killed more cows than tuberculosis did, but fortunately it is not transmissible to human beings, as tuberculosis is, and so for a great many years no official measures were taken to bring about its elimination. It was quite incurable and was spread from cow to cow by infected grazing.

The Ministry of Agriculture (Animal Health Division) some years ago set about eliminating bovine tuberculosis by the method of tuberculin testing all the cattle in the country and slaughtering affected cows. They were ably assisted in this task by the practising veterinary surgeons acting as local veterinary inspectors. The result was that in 1961, the country was declared free of bovine tuberculosis, a great achievement for which the veterinary profession was entirely responsible. Tuberculin testing, on a smaller scale, will be continued for years in case from some source or another infection should be reintroduced.

Before tuberculin testing was enforced throughout the country, the Tuberculosis Order demanded that farmers should report cows which were coughing and showing signs of tuberculosis, those which were affected with tuberculosis of the udder—and therefore giving tuberculous milk, which would infect children and possibly adults. They were also required to report cases of emaciation in cattle arising from tuberculosis. These were cases in which the cow had been tuberculous, probably for years, had reached almost the point of death, and had already done most of the damage she was ever likely to do.

The greatest good the Tuberculosis Order ever did was in getting rid of some—admittedly a small proportion—of the cows which were yielding milk containing living, active tubercle bacilli, which was hitherto being distributed for human consumption in the raw state.

Before the pasteurisation and sterilisation of milk came into general use large numbers of children died every year from bovine tubercle, while out of the hundreds or thousands which became infected but remained alive, a great many became crippled for life from joint tuberculosis.

For some reason the immense danger which was incurred by drinking unboiled, unsterilised, or unpasteurised milk was never really impressed upon public mentality and it is unlikely that the majority of parents had the least idea of the dangers to which their children were exposed when given raw milk to drink.

It was even the custom to send country children to the farms at milking time to fetch jugfuls of milk "warm from the cow," in the peculiar belief that such a beverage imparted strength and well-being!

It would be true to say that never at any time prior to the elimination of bovine tuberculosis was the alarming incidence of the disease in cattle and its possible effects on children, impressed upon parents as it should have been.

Another source of danger was the "household cow," the animal kept on farms and by country households, to supply milk for the family. Such cows were seldom tested and not infrequently were tuberculous and may have been yielding tubercle infected milk.

I was staying in a village near the Scottish border a few years ago and I was given particulars of an incident which shows the good that has been done by the veterinary profession in ridding our dairy herds of this disease, undoubtedly one of the greatest evils so far as public health was concerned.

The following is the story of only one case but it is typical of what was happening to other human families throughout the country.

A lady, a widow with one girl of eight years, stayed at a hotel near the Border for health reasons after losing her husband in a car accident. The hotel was very isolated and depended, during the season, upon anglers who congregated for the trout and salmon fishing. Finding the place lonely out-of-season, the lady persuaded another lady with a daughter of the same age as her own, to spend part of the year with them at the hotel.

The proprietor kept two cows. Neither of these had been tested, and they supplied milk and cream for the guests. The children had the greater part of the cream and were given the milk, raw and warm, to drink daily. One of these cows must have suffered from tuberculosis of the udder.

Both children contracted bovine tubercle. One died; the other was left with a chronic tubercular arthritis from which there was little hope of recovery. This case was probed to its source and the infection definitely traced to one cow.

But how many thousands of children throughout the land became infected from bulk milk taken from a large number of cows and mixed together, will never be fully disclosed.

The reason that cows continue to undergo further tests after the country has been declared free of bovine tuberculosis is that cows which are in an advanced stage of the disease without showing typical or obvious symptoms, may not react to the tuberculin test. In addition, some skin reactions to intradermal tuberculin may be due not to tubercle but to a non-specific infection introduced by birds or small field animals, and these infections are not generally dangerous to human beings.

Human tubercle, carried by farm workers, may also produce reactions, but cows do not develop the human disease, although human beings are susceptible to the disease taken from the cow.

Another cause of a crop of reactions in an apparently tubercle-free herd may arise from a broken drainpipe carrying human sewage, allowing it to permeate the soil of the field in which cattle are grazing.

The Animal Health Division of the Ministry of Agriculture, under the capable and energetic leadership of Sir John Ritchie,

Chief Veterinary Officer, as well as the many hundreds of local veterinary inspectors, deserve the thanks of the British public for this determined and successful attempt to eradicate bovine tuberculosis from our herds. Not only will the success of this enterprise prevent wastage and loss of cattle and dairy produce, but it will also ensure the safety of all milk foods in this respect, and undoubtedly it will save countless human lives, especially those of children, and preserve a great many more from crippledom.

Until the disease was eradicated among cattle, in spite of the Tuberculosis Order which so often was disregarded, there was a marked laxity on the part of the farmer in notifying the presence of disease in his herd. Cases of udder infection continued to be milked so long as the milk could be sold, even if this necessitated mixing it with the milk from other cows. This may have been due partly to ignorance and partly to lack of understanding of the consequences to human life and health arising from the consumption of tuberculous milk.

The following provides an example:

Some years after I had set up in practice I visited on behalf of the Ministry of Agriculture, a cow reported by her owner as a suspected case of tuberculosis. This poor animal had reached the stage when it lay on the ground, a mere skeleton covered by skin, entirely unable to rise. Not only did this prove to be a case of generalised tuberculosis but the cow had a grossly affected udder and her milk was found, microscopically, to be teeming with tubercle bacilli.

The cow was destroyed and the carcase taken away for post-mortem examination. A week later I met the owner when I was inspecting a cattle market. He commenced the usual lengthy lamentation concerned mainly with the small sum which was to be awarded him by way of compensation for his cow. I think that in reality he was more grieved at losing the price of the small amount of milk the cow had yielded right up to her end.

"Don't think," he said to me, "that it's only the loss of the cow I'm worried about. I'm more distressed about that poor little child down at the post office. You see, her mother, would never have any milk for her except what came from the old Guernsey you took from me. That milk suited the child, and believe me, she's going to miss it more than another kiddie would.

You see, she's been delicate—since birth!"

Of course all our clients are not quite so innocent as this one was; in fact some are very artful, especially in connection with calling in the veterinary surgeon in some case which may lead to litigation.

I was asked on one occasion to visit a cow by a person I would have had no hesitation in describing, when first I met her, as a "dear old lady."

She carried on, with help from outside, a small farm in an out-of-the-way neighbourhood. When I arrived at the farm in this hill country she explained to me why she wanted me. She had recently sold "one of her best cows" to a local farmer with the verbal warranty common to the district, that she was "right and straight," meaning that she was sound. On getting the cow home it appeared that the purchaser had other ideas as to the interpretation of the term, as a result of which he wrote the lady asking for the return of the purchase price, in exchange for the cow.

Apparently he recieved no acknowledgement of his letter with the result that a week later, when the old lady came down from bed, she found a cow tied by a halter to her front gate.

As is usual a veterinary surgeon, unfortunately myself in this instance, was called in to decide who was right on the question of the cow's soundness, with the certainty of making one enemy for life, if not two.

"He says," she explained, "that this cow has a bad quarter and that he ain't a-going to keep her, and the dirty blackguard brought her back and left her hitched on the gate while I was fast in my bed, asleep.

"Now I want you to write me a certificate and say she is right and straight in all respects and I can then send him a copy of it."

I made a brief examination and it was perfectly obvious the cow had an indurated hind quarter with involvement of the supramammary gland.

I took a sample of milk for examination and this subsequently proved positive for the presence of tubercle bacilli.

I pointed out to the old lady that I suspected the presence of mammary tuberculosis and that until I had examined the milk sample the cow must be placed in isolation. To my complete surprise she took the news quite well.

"Isn't her milk fit to drink?" she asked.

"Certainly not, or at least not until I have tested the sample."

She made no more ado about it but commenced to regale me with a long discourse regarding the general excellence of her herd while I was on my way to inspect them as a part of my duty. Her other cows all looked healthy and well, and, as I told her, were a credit to her good management. I probably laid the praise on fairly thick as matters between us seemed to be going pretty well and I wanted them to stay that way.

It crossed my mind what a coincidence it was that she had attempted to sell the only obviously unhealthy cow in the herd, but I made no comment on this point.

The lady then insisted that I see her dairy, of which she seemed very proud, and although it was no part of my duty to visit it, I consented with good grace.

Everything in the dairy was clean and tidy and thoroughly up-to-date.

I was about to wish her good day when she suggested I might care for a glass of milk.

In the usual way I am not very fond of long draughts of milk, but the morning was passing, lunch was a long way ahead, and as I wanted to remain on good terms with the lady, I accepted.

She drew off half-a-pint from a can which I imagined contained her very best sample. Slowly I drank it down.

"Did you enjoy it?" she asked.

"Yes. Very much," I answered, perhaps a little untruthfully.

"And you wouldn't think there was much wrong with my herd if that was a sample of the milk from it?"

"Certainly not," I replied.

"Well," she remarked, "I'm glad to hear you say so. You see

that can of milk and the glassful you swallowed, came from the cow you examined!"

In my early days a great many of the minor illnesses of cattle were grouped together under the diagnosis of "indigestion." Of late years a deal of stress has been laid upon certain metabolic diseases and of these the condition of ketosis, known generally in dairy circles as *acetonaemia* has been the one most often recorded. To the man with a "nose," the smell carried by the breath of the affected cow as well as her urine, is highly reminiscent of the old-fashioned peardrops, a feature of cattle about which poets have sung, quite unaware that it was merely a sign of illness.

However it is treated nowadays by a combination of cortisone and glucose, which after all is not so very different to the treatment of "indigestion" years ago when cows were dosed with carbonate of ammonia and nux vomica in powder form, given twice daily *with one to two pounds of treacle.* The only difference is that the old folk discovered how to cure the disease before they had discovered its cause.

I must confess, however, that since the new boys in the profession set to work on bovine research, they have made a number of important discoveries with the result that the present generation knows a great deal more about cows than my own generation did.

A disease which has plagued cattle from time immemorial, and continues to do so in these more enlightened times, is contagious abortion. In my own experience in Cornwall, very few farms forty years ago were free of the disease and it was the custom for one heifer or young cow out of every three to give birth to her calf from the sixth to seventh month of gestation instead of carrying it a full nine months. Most abortions occurred at the seventh month and curiously quite a number of calves born at this period lived, while those born at eight months almost always died.

But cows which went the full nine months and delivered apparently healthy calves might still be carriers of the disease.

It was difficult, strange as it may seem, to convince farmers, years ago, that the condition was spread from cow to cow. They were sure it was due to the growth of a fungus, ergot, on the grass and cereals. Their method of combating the disease was to include a Billy goat in the herd. The goat acted as a mascot and usually headed the herd and led the cows from place to place on the farm.

Farmers were quite certain that the goat proceeding in front of the cows, ate the ergot off the grass and in this way saved the cows that would have consumed it from aborting as a consequence.

Other people were equally convinced that the smell of the Billy goat, apparent from a long distance when the wind blew in the right direction, drove away all the germs, which could not face up to it.

Contagious abortion seems to descend upon a herd in waves, a lot of abortions occurred, followed by a period of apparent freedom, then by another batch. It is a self-limiting disease in the sense that only about half the cows which abort do so a second time, while only a quarter of those which abort twice do so a third time. The result is that the older cows may appear to possess an immunity. It was this age immunity no doubt which was responsible for the apparent cleverness of the Billy goat.

Unfortunately heifers, brought into the herd, were devoid of immunity, and the Billy goat was powerless to do anything to help them.

But the Ministry of Agriculture with the assistance of its local veterinary inspectors, have decided that having eliminated tuberculosis from the herds they will now set about clearing them of contagious abortion also by the free use of their live vaccine known as S.19. Injected into young female calves this produces a considerable degree of immunity. The result of earlier inoculations has been so encouraging that a scheme is now afoot to vaccinate *all* female calves and it seems that within a few years this great scourge will be eradicated and it will probably stay away so long as vaccination is continued.

The service replaces the existing Calfhood Vaccination Scheme from May 1st. 1962, and the estimated cost of vaccine for the first year is £15,500. Last year (1961) under the original scheme 436,309 vaccinations were carried out costing the farmers 2/6 each.

A Ministry spokesman said that at present about 2 per cent of all pregnancies in cattle end in abortion and a quarter of these were due to contagious abortion. A Ministry survey on abortion is being carried out and will be published in 1962.

This means that the veterinary profession will have conquered another of the diseases which has helped not only to keep farmers poor but to limit the milk supply available to the public.

But in some ways this is not the most important aspect of the elimination of this disease.

Bovine contagious abortion organisms known as brucella are excreted in the milk of the affected cow and when milk from such animals is consumed by human beings it frequently gives rise to a febrile disease known as undulant fever.

This disease assumes a number of forms in men and women.

The ordinary type is a relapsing fever, somewhat influenza-like apart from the fact that there are fairly frequent rises and falls of body temperature, which may persist for weeks or months. Not every case of this disease prevents the patient from getting up and moving about, but it causes headache and weakness, together with depression.

In other instances pains in joints are experienced, and both in animals and man many patients suffering from arthritic conditions are found to harbour abortion bacilli in their joints.

Veterinary surgeons are very frequent sufferers from the disease. Infection can take place through the skin, and as during obstetrical operations and especially when removing the retained membranes from cows which have calved prematurely and failed to discharge them, their hands and arms are soaked in the infected uterine fluids, very few country practitioners escape. A good many of those who do not develop active febrile symptoms exhibit persistent skin rashes, a form of allergy which become more severe whenever the hands and arms are introduced into the vagina of an infected cow.

Ordinary members of the public who do not handle, or even go near cattle, used to develop undulant fever from drinking raw milk, but since the bulk of the milk has been subjected to heat treatment by pasteurisation, or sterilisation, the incidence of the disease has been less.

Although occasionally doctors take samples of human blood for agglutination tests in suspected cases, it is likely that more cases of the disease escape detection than are diagnosed, since in many instances the symptoms shown may easily be overlooked or confused with some other disease such as influenza.

A considerable percentage of the human population of many countries shows an enhanced titre to brucella infection, often without being aware of having ever suffered from undulant fever, but the incidence is less since the pasterisation and sterilisation of milk became general.

It is to be hoped that the present attempt on the part of the profession to stamp out the disease among cattle will be successful, and that at the same time it will put an end to the wholesale infection of human beings.

Another disease which people may contract from birds and animals is parrot fever, known as *psittacosis*. It receives this name since it is present in the psittacine birds, the parrots, budgerigars and their like, in which it still persists in this country.

It may also occur in other birds which congregate in flocks, such as pigeons, starlings, sparrows, puffins, eider ducks, seagulls and gannets. It is spread by roosting in close proximity, and among birds other than the parrot family, it is known as ornithosis.

It would seem that the organism which causes the disease varies considerably in its potency. When human beings develop the disease through contact with sick parrots and budgerigars, the effects are serious and in some outbreaks the mortality rate is high. But pigeons and other birds carry a similar disease very frequently of seemingly lower virulence, and although pigeon fanciers have sometimes become infected from their birds, the mortality rate is much lower generally than in psittacosis from parrots or budgerigars.

The organism may, however, undergo what is known as mutation, a change in its nature and in its degree of virulence. It could then happen that the pigeons in the Square, which the children feed and allow to settle upon them, might convey a serious type of undulating fever with pneumonic complications. The danger, even today, arising from sick budgerigars, frequent carriers of this dangerous disease, is realised by very few people who keep these birds.

It is quite likely that far more cases of psittacosis occur in humans than are ever diagnosed.

Some thirty-odd years ago, a very serious outbreak of psittacosis occurred in England from disease in imported parrots. So severe was it and so high the human mortality that for a great many years after, the importation of parrots was prohibited.

I, myself, contracted the disease during this outbreak since I included the inspection of the animals kept in a private zoo in my daily round.

The proprietors purchased several dozen finches from a well-known firm of importers. When these arrived by rail, packed in quite a small box, it was found when it was unpacked and opened that about half-a-dozen birds lay dead on the floor.

Not knowing sufficient about birds, I attributed this to lack of air and overcrowding, but when we wrote a complaint to the firm, we were assured that this was the correct way to pack small birds as the risk from overcrowding was less than that from having too much space which would permit wing-flapping and injury.

The surviving birds were scattered about the zoo in cages, and about a fortnight later, more had died. Then a creature of the anteater family became ill and died. Out of a dozen flying squirrels all but two collapsed on the floor of their cage and died. So did a fox and a badger, then more birds of various kinds. Finally the monkeys began to sicken. I made post-mortems on all these animals without discovering the real cause of the illness. It must be remembered that little was known about psittacosis in this country at that time.

One small squirrel monkey, Bimbo, used to run free about the grounds. He always met me at the entrance, took hold of my hand and walked around the zoo with me every morning. When the monkeys began to sicken, I noticed that Bimbo seemed poorly and disinclined to walk. Instead, he climed onto my shoulder. This did not please the other monkeys, or those well enough to signify their disapproval, and I tried to get him down. The result was that he bit me in the lobe of the left ear, not savagely but hard enough to draw blood. I do not know whether this infected me or if I became contaminated from making post-mortems.

After a few days I began to get inordinately sleepy and would doze off, sometimes in the middle of a conversation. On the ninth morning after being bitten I awoke at 3 a.m. filled with intense exhilaration. I cannot describe the feeling. I think it must have been a foretaste of Heaven for I was extremely happy and had never felt so well in my life. I felt as though my body was floating in space, delightfully warm and comfortable.

Five hours later, I awoke with an intense headache and could not open my eyes to face the daylight.

From then on, I grew worse daily. My temperature went up gradually to 104°F. every six hours then fell to 98.5° and repeated the process quite regularly at the same intervals. Patches of pneumonia came and went, usually in one lung at a time, sometimes in both.

On the twenty-first day of my illness a friend called to see me. He found me on my hands and knees in bed, struggling to breathe.

Very shaken, he adjourned to a nearby hostel to seek consolation, and there he met a reporter from the local newspaper. Whether it was the consoling effect of the alcohol or a plain misunderstanding I do not know, but my friend intimated to the reporter that I would be dead by the next morning. This was good enough for the newsmonger.

At noon on the following day the paper printed a full-length obituary notice, several columns of it as real news happened to be scarce, in which my career, true and fictitious, received the fullest attention.

When the account was read to me, I decided that any soul so pure, so indispensable and so imbued with all the virtues ascribed to it by that young reporter, was far too valuable to succumb to parrot trouble.

A few hours later when the wreaths began to arrive and I lay in bed surrounded by them with a particularly sweet white specimen adorning my head as a halo, I felt so amused and enlivened that I took a distinct turn for the better.

However, it was another twelve months before I shook off the asthmatical and paralytic complications, but that I survived all these is now evident.

In Central Africa, until recent years, one of the customs of the chief of a tribe was to send to a chief of another tribe (whom he did not like), a present of gaudy parrot feathers packed in leaves. The feathers were taken from a parrot found dead in the forest. It is said that in many instances the recipient who unpacked the feathers and possibly wore them, frequently died. This was always cited as an example of native black magic, but it is by no means impossible that the bird from which the feathers were obtained may have died from psittacosis which is prevalent among parrots in the wild state.

Speaking of zoological collections and of monkeys prompts me, for security reasons, to make a brief mention of a disease common in monkeys which assumes little importance in the monkey but is easily transmitted to human beings, and causes a disease which is practically 100 per cent fatal.

Not many people handle monkeys or come close to them excepting in a zoo, but occasionally young specimens are purchased as pets, often for children, and although, as one who has kept a lot of monkeys, I would not recommend one as a pet for a variety of reasons, this particular disease danger is something quite different and far more serious than bitten fingers.

Since very large numbers of monkeys have been crowded into cages and imported by air for the purpose of preparing poliomyelitis vaccine to vaccinate children against "polio," a disease has been recognised in them, spread rapidly by contact on the air journey. It is a form of monkey herpes not unlike the type we get on our lips after a common cold.

In monkeys it is caused by a virus, known now as "Simian virus B." The human herpes simplex lives within our bodies and gives rise to a lip or facial eruption, when our resistance has been lowered by some other virus infection, (cf, the common cold).

Men become infected by handling these recently imported monkeys, or from bites, although direct contact with a facial lesion on a monkey may be sufficient to convey infection.

The wound or infected skin area becomes swollen and surrounded by small vesicles. Between ten and twenty days after the bite, an acute infection of the brain (encephalomyelitis) develops, followed by coma and early death. So far, out of the cases which have been diagnosed, only one person has recovered.

Herpes B is a natural parasite of monkeys and as many as 27 per cent of animals in a monkey colony may carry the disease. The incidence may increase to 75 per cent under crowded conditions. Very few monkeys show any illness apart from the facial eruption.

As monkey tissues are used to prepare pools of virus for the manufacture of poliomyelitis vaccine, the importance of detecting the presence of virus B is at once apparent.

About 1 per cent of virus pools have been known to carry the virus, a fact which makes it necessary to destroy them.

As I have mentioned already, most of the local veterinary surgeons in country areas, who carry on their own practices, act as local veterinary inspectors to the Animal Health Division of the Ministry of Agriculture and Fisheries. In areas where the cattle population is considerable certain assistants in the practices may also be appointed. The notifiable diseases of animals which come under veterinary control are:

Rinderpest or Cattle Plague	Pleuro Poneumonia (Contagious)
Foot and Mouth Disease	Anthrax
Sheep Scab	Rabies
Sheep Pox	Epizootic Lymphangitis
Glanders of Farcy	Parasitic Mange
Swine Fever	Tuberculosis
Fowl Pox	Fowl Pest

Collectively, these provide a lot of work for the veterinary surgeon and during the past few years tuberculin testing alone has taken a very important place in almost every practice.

Preventive medicine is regarded very highly in this country, and cattle, pigs, sheep, dogs and cats, are vaccinated against numerous diseases.

One serious omission from the activities of the veterinary profession is that meat, which nearly everyone eats, is not examined before or after slaughter by qualified veterinary surgeons in the great majority of cases, but only by lay meat inspectors. This is no aspersion upon a very useful, hard-working and competent body of men. There is no doubt whatever that they do a splendid job to the extent of their knowledge, but unlike the qualified veterinary surgeon they are not trained pathologists. Although there is no reason why these regular meat inspectors should not continue to operate, it is also quite certain that they should do so under veterinary supervision so that doubtful carcases could receive expert examination with microscopic and bacteriological tests when required. Meat is so important a food that the public should be completely guarded against possible disease.

It is true that a few of the larger abattoirs in England, and probably a higher percentage in Scotland and Northern Ireland, come under veterinary supervision, but the bulk of the smaller abattoirs through which by far the greater portion of all meat for human consumption passes, are entirely devoid of qualified veterinary supervision. It must be confessed that veterinary surgeons are already a very overworked body of men but the number of graduates could be increased if meat inspection were to be carried out under veterinary supervision.

This lack of professional meat inspection is a crying disgrace to our country and a matter in which we lag behind the majority of civilised countries throughout the world.

There is of course another angle, the economic one. Veterinary surgeons would demand considerably higher salaries than lay inspectors. This might result in a very small increase in the price of meat and it is a question whether the public would be prepared to consider this as a worthwhile insurance against the possible transmission of disease to themselves and their families.

On the other hand, veterinary inspection of meat would provide a valuable index of the existence of disease and its origin. This would be an additional safeguard. Veterinary examination would also provide material (now completely wasted) which would help considerably the study of pathology, and would be of considerable value in studying the causation and nature of certain diseases, not only to the veterinary profession but also to the medical profession.

Chapter Five

HORSE PRACTICE

IN CONTRAST with the present day, horse practice as I knew it from 1909 onwards, and in my schooldays before that date, provided a very great part of our work. Horses were everywhere, both in town and country, and just as lock-up garages now appear in every nook and corner, so did stables in every large town. In most cases they were an important part of the premises and usually were quite close to the dwelling house, the original idea being that horses if not always in sight, should always be within sound, in case one got cast in the night or developed an attack of colic which caused it to throw itself about in its loose box.

Horses of all kinds were required; for riding, hunting, driving, light and heavy delivery work in towns and country; ploughing, harvesting, carting and general farm work on the land. This meant, of course, that horses were frequently changing hands, just as cars do today, the difference being that there were few "new" horses apart from freshly broken horses not yet suitable for town work. Most of the horses were secondhand or thirdhand as the case might be, and no horse of reasonable age depreciated a hundred pounds every year as a car does; in fact from four years to eight years old, most horses increased in value so long as they remained sound. Practically every horse sold was examined for soundness by a veterinary surgeon employed by the prospective purchaser. This examination was—and still is—a rather protracted proceeding, usually occupying an hour of the veterinary surgeon's time.

It was always carried out in a very precise and orthodox manner and very great attention was paid to even the most minute details. The examination for soundness became such an exact performance and the confidence placed in the veterinary examiner so complete, that a new word came into the English language, the verb "to vet."

All important propositions and agreements, nowadays have to

be "vetted," which means they must be given thorough examination by an authority of the highest competence and integrity.

The examination of a horse necessitated the veterinary surgeon visiting the animal in its own stable, since exercising the horse or taking it to the premises of the veterinary surgeon caused it to be moved, which might sometimes lessen or completely remove signs of lameness which the horse might show if it were brought out of its stable and examined in what was termed the "cold" state.

With this in mind many veterinary surgeons refused to name an hour for their visits to dealers and sellers, as knowing the horse was to be examined at a certain time they would see that it was exercised, "warmed up" and back in its box, before the hour when the veterinary surgeon was due to put in an appearance.

Dealers used to practice all manner of tricks to attempt to hoodwink the veterinary surgeon, though I am afraid it was often a waste of time as the "vets" learned most of these tricks at an early stage of their career, and it was not easy to devise fresh ones. Their idea was that if they could deceive the veterinary surgeon and induce him to pass a horse as sound, the responsibility would fall upon the veterinary surgeon, if the horse proved unsound shortly afterwards, rather than upon the seller.

A common trick when a horse had "spavined hocks," one larger on the inside than the other, was to tap the sound hock repeatedly with a small wooden mallet to produce swelling so that the two hocks matched each other. Horses affected with spavin always go better, and less lame in their hocks, the further they travel.

The dealer after using his little mallet, would tie the horse in the yard on a halter, and set one or two boys to groom it. Whenever nobody was looking they had to make the horse keep turning over from one side to the other, without untying it. This kept the hocks supple and lessened their stiffness, and at the same time might deceive the veterinary surgeon on his arrival into believing the horse had stood for a considerable while quite still in one place while being groomed.

Cracks in the hoofs would be neatly filled with hot sealing wax of an appropriate colour, then well polished with hoof blacking.

When tendons were contracted or "bowed," the veterinary

surgeon would be told, with many apologies, that as he was not expected, the horse had been left running out in the field, where it would be found with thick mud reaching up to the knees and hocks. Unless one insisted on an immediate application of the horsepipe to its limbs such infirmities might easily go unnoticed.

When a horse was "gone in its wind," it would be dosed with arsenic in small doses over a long period, or given a pound of small shot by mixing it with food, or by stirring it into thick gruel and administering it as a drench. The pound of shot lying in the stomach was reputed to bring temporary improvement, which might hoodwink the veterinary surgeon carrying out the examination.

If the horse was known to be slightly lame, the owner or attendant would rush it out of the box, run it completely out of sight, then come back walking slowly, the man complaining that "his rheumatics hurt him cruel," and he was quite unable to run the horse up again. Then, on occasion, another trick would be tried out.

If the dealer were aware that the horse was a little lame, say in the left fore foot, he might find a conveniently shaped small stone before the veterinary surgeon arrived. He would then hammer this stone firmly between the horse's frog and the inner branch of the shoe.

When the horse was trotted up and the veterinary surgeon remarked upon the lameness, the dealer would put on a surprised look, then searching the foot, would "find" the stone jammed in place.

After this had been removed with some difficulty, the dealer would apologise, saying that no doubt the stone had caused some temporary lameness which would probably disappear by the following day.

If the veterinary surgeon happened to be young and inexperienced, he might accept this as the truth, but the older examiners would have learned this trick, and probably others of its kind.

A few dealers made a practice of buying lame horses for little money, and having them "unnerved." This operation involved section of the nerve (such as the plantar nerve) which lay between the seat of lameness and the brain. After such an operation the horse felt no pain and travelled sound, but at a later date it might suddenly cast off the entire wall of the foot, or the pedal bone might penetrate the sole, so that the animal would have to be destroyed.

It was by no means easy in every case to discover the seat of such an operation (neurectomy) but every veterinary surgeon in those days carried a pin stuck in the lapel of his jacket, and with this he used to test the horse's coronets to ensure they had sensation and were responsive to pin prick.

It was not unusual for the veterinary surgeon to examine one or several horses every day of the week, with the exception of Sunday, when it was considered illegal (whether rightly or wrongly I never discovered) to examine a horse, or even to sell one.

On a market day he might be kept busy examining horses. All these, of course, would already have been "warmed-up," before he saw them, and any slight lameness shown when the horse was "cold," might have been minimised. But in every case the competent veterinary surgeon after completing his examination and finding nothing abnormal, would insist on the horse being shut in a loose box or tied up in a stall for half-an-hour, after which it would be again brought out and run up for further inspection.

All horses, during their examination, had to be galloped to enable the veterinary surgeon to test their "wind." In our own market town this was done, in the absence of a grass field, by galloping each horse a quarter of a mile up a very steep hill just outside the market premises.

To enable the examination to be carried out without undue noise or interruption it was usual to send one man to the bottom of the hill and another to the top, to stop all the traffic, until the test had been completed. Needless to say, the veterinary surgeon himself had also to negotiate the quarter of a mile up the steep hill each time he examined a horse!

One of the evils which has been done away with by legislation, to the delight of every veterinary surgeon, is the operation of "docking."

Until a few years ago, practically all horses other than Thoroughbreds, had all but six inches of their tail removed by operation.

The instrument used to sever the tail, much thicker than a man's wrist, was a kind of guillotine, operated by two hands so that a semicircular knife was forced into a similar shaped cavity into which the tail of the horse was fitted. This barbarous operation was certainly carried out either under local or epidural anaesthesia, but the haemorrhage was severe and could only be controlled sufficiently rapidly by searing the bleeding tail with a specially shaped iron made red-hot in a fire.

Searing seems a crude method, but in reality it was the most efficient, since the stump of the tail of a carthorse is quite three inches in diameter and the rush of blood through it was so powerful that ligation was too slow a method.

The docking knife was hinged at its extremity and great strength was required to bring the two handles together and close the knife upon the tail so as to cut through it in a single stroke.

It must be remembered also that to prevent any risk of breaking the back of a heavy carthorse by casting it and administering an anaesthetic, the operation was almost invariably performed with the horse standing. The operator was then stationed at the kicking end of the horse, close behind its two hind feet and directly in the line of fire. The operation was one attended always by considerable danger to the veterinary surgeon.

I have particularly vivid recollections of docking a huge, five-year-old Shire stallion. This was at any time sufficiently dangerous for the operator, but in this particular case an additional risk made its appearance, and it certainly materialised.

The stallion was a rather evil-natured beast at its best. He was to be shown, and for this purpose had in those days to be docked, an operation which should have been carried out when he was only a few days old.

As he was not the kind of animal anyone would wish to stand behind in a loose box, it was decided that the operation would have to be performed outside the stable where there was room to escape his heels.

Unfortunately, however, outside meant on the village green,

onto which the stable opened. There was no other space in this somewhat built-up area. We would have adjourned to a field but we were compelled to remain close to the kitchen fire in which the irons were to be heated to sear the tail after the amputation.

We chose an early hour in the morning when we thought the Square would be empty of people, but in a village news travels very speedily and even before the operation commenced a small crowd had gathered in gloating anticipation. There were all kinds of people. Shopping seemed to have commenced early for many carried bags, while the shop girls and young men employed in the neighbourhood, and even a number of children were all on the scene. The only person absent seems to have been the village constable. It was certainly an ideal day for a little sightseeing, a warm day in early August with the sun streaming down upon us. Even the horse appeared to be enjoying himself up to this stage.

I had clipped and scrubbed the root of the tail and injected the local anaesthetic, and I stood there waiting for it to take effect, a little self-conscious in front of that growing crowd I fear, for I was still very young and inordinately shy.

I held the heavy guillotine in position, my two hands grasping the handles, my arms widespread and my whole attention now focussed upon that swift, strong stroke which would chop instantaneously through that thick tail and leave the free portion in the hands of one of the onlookers, who had volunteered to draw gently upon the cotton rope I had attached to the hair at its lower extremity.

I took a deep breath, prepared to bring down the knife—and then it happened! I recollect taking one fleeting glance around to make sure I had space behind me to retreat from those massive hind hoofs, and thinking to myself that the village maidens, clustering rather too closely around me, must be of the school that delights in bloodshed.

My arm was about to descend to make the stroke; a girl gave a quick gasp of anticipation, and a particularly vivacious bee descended beneath the neckband of my shirt and stung me on the chest. From there, in the fraction of a second, it migrated downwards to more vulnerable portions of my anatomy and set up a veritable barrage with its sting.

I had been standing there in my shirt, trousers and braces.

The agony was unendurable.

I did not hesitate to take immediate action. I will spare you the shocking details. Suffice it to say that a second later, bereft of braces and trousers, I was running madly across that village green seeking the haven of the stallion's loose box.

Some of the men doubled up with laughter, some stood gaping with mouths wide open. The village maidens uttered shrill screams, whether from delight or horror I cannot say.

The horse alone was completely unmoved by all that went on around him.

Nevertheless, for sometime afterwards my fame as an acrobatic surgeon persisted, and whenever it was noised abroad that I was to perform another, or similar operation, I would find the utmost difficulty in preserving complete privacy.

It was the custom in my father's practice, in which I grew up, to open wide the large double gates of the surgery yard at 2 p.m., excepting on Sundays. In would troop a miscellaneous collection of horses, of all sizes and breeds. Quite often there would be a few donkeys among them, since practically every Cornish miner travelled to the mine and home again seated in a two-wheeled shay, usually painted bright red or blue or yellow, drawn by his donkey.

The shay was always spotlessly clean and there were two main types. Each consisted of a pair of shafts which were extended backwards to give attachment to an axle and a pair of wheels, and a seat consisting of a six-inch board stretched from shaft to shaft.

The difference between the two types of shay lay in the wheels. One kind had 2 ordinary bicycle wheels with pneumatic tyres; the other had large buggy wheels, very light in make, four or five feet high with either flat iron tyres, or solid rubber tyres.

On the wooden seat the driver reposed with his two feet resting on the donkey's rump.

Nobody, in these days, can have any idea of the quality and the fiery natures of those Cornish donkeys. Their owners worshipped them, and the donkeys used to walk into the kitchens and even sleep in them. They were always closely clipped and their thin hides were smooth and brushed until they shone like the skin of a Thoroughbred stallion. Occasionally a miner drove a mare donkey but the majority were males and entire.

They were like a Thoroughbred, or possibly more like an Arab, in other ways. They would be fairly docile until harnessed, and as soon as the shafts descended over their backs they would rear and struggle to be away. They travelled all the time, whether on the hard roads or on grass, at full gallop, and quite a fast gallop at that. It was surprising how far they could gallop without getting winded or weary. Nobody who has seen only the Irish donkeys or those on an English beach can have any realisation of the activity, agility and endurance of a well-fed, well-groomed donkey.

The local agricultural shows always put on classes, chariot races in reality for donkeys; usually one class for stallions and one for mares. They were, judged for conformation and speed. The number of entries was enormous and it was seldom that the showring was large enough to give freedom to all competitors.

They were driven always on long reins and at the start of each race, the drivers had to stand four feet behind the shay, reins in hand.

When the flag dropped each donkey reared high into the air, took a flying leap forward and was away at full gallop. Each driver had to run behind and vault into his seat while the donkey was galloping. One well-known competitor who entered his turn-out at nearly every show walked on two crutches, and yet he used to follow on these, haul himself and his crutches aboard; and the remarkable thing is that he almost invariably ended in the first three.

The course was four circuits of the ring with nothing barred. If one competitor could not get ahead of the other the object was to turn over his shay, either by direct collision or by locking the wheels of the two vehicles until one capsized. All this was accompanied by wild shouting on the part of the drivers and a tumult of cheers and exhortations from the ringside.

I think the spectators regarded the two donkey races which followed the jumping and usually concluded the show, as the most exciting part of the proceedings.

I remember a certain very well-known horseman coming from the Midlands to judge the horses at a Cornish show and being asked also to judge the donkeys. He had never met Cornish donkeys before and was amazed at their quality and their lively dispositions.

Then came the donkey races in harness. The judge stood well in front of the long line of donkeys waiting to drop his flag, imagining no doubt from his previous experience of donkeys that he had lots of time to get out of the way. But these were Cornish donkeys.

The moment his flag descended, every donkey reared into the air and about thirty donkeys and shays took one flying leap over the judge's head.

We picked him up and got him to the side of the ring before they began the second circuit, but he was badly shaken, though not injured.

Some thirty years later I met this gentleman again and he assured me that he was never so surprised in the whole of his life as when he dropped his flag at a Cornish show.

But to return to our yardful of horses.

Most of those which came in during our afternoon sessions were surgical cases, recovering after operation, preparing for operation, or cases of lameness requiring diagnosis and treatment.

Firing joints and tendons, under local or general anaesthesia, by burning a pattern, usually herringbone; or driving needle-like points into the skin over joints, by means of sharp or pointed irons, made red hot; was a common treatment years ago, and is practised even today as it appears to produce better and more lasting results than more modern physiotherapy. It is true that the irons are less often heated in the fire, and that the operation is more frequently carried out by electrical thermo-cautery.

To a certain extent this old treatment has given way to low-wave therapy, but it still has a great many advocates.

Whether physiotherapy or the actual application of hot irons produces the good results, or if the enforced idleness following the actual cautery is of more service than the active treatment given, is still a matter of conjecture.

As a rule, without the firing, the rest would never materialise.

A large number of horses came into our hospital to be operated upon for poll-evil, fistulous withers, shoulder tumours, capped elbows and quittor.

The ubiquitous shoulder tumour, quite benign and caused by infection rubbed into the skin, eventually reaching the biceps muscle, grew very quickly, often to a great size before being presented for treatment.

In the course of our daily rounds we attended numerous cases of bowel impaction and bowel displacements in horses. Owing to the peculiar disposition and the immense size of the horse's large intestine and caecum, the suffering of these patients was intense, and they had to be controlled throughout by injections of morphia and doses of chloral hydrate to prevent them throwing themselves about and inflicting injury upon themselves and their attendants.

Influenza and strangles used to make their appearance every summer and spread by putting horses in hotel stables in the same way that we now park cars; and also by public drinking troughs.

Influenza was much like the same disease in man, but strangles was more akin to a severe type of quinsy in which abscesses developed and needed lancing in the throat and facial regions, and sometimes in other glands in any part of the body, also in the lungs and liver.

Every Monday morning we used to be called out to see cases of lymphangitis, known better as "Monday morning leg," in which a leg became swollen and its glands inflamed as a result of the horse standing, often on full diet, all the week-end in the stable.

Other horses from the same cause developed laminitis, or "fever in the feet," which made it difficult for them to stand. Years ago this was a protracted disease which often led to crippling and eventually to destruction. More recently it has been found to be an allergic condition and to respond rapidly and dramatically to injection of an antihistamine. Hydrocortisone injections nowadays have a similar effect—or would do so if we had the horses.

Another common disease was known as periodic ophthalmia, which was recurrent and ended usually in blindness.

Horse practice, alas, has almost completely disappeared, apart from in certain districts where hunters, polo ponies, show jumpers, flatracers and steeple-chasers are still fairly plentiful.

On a market day every available yard and stable was packed

with the traps and horses which conveyed the farmer, his wife, and sometimes his family, to market, and to see a little "high life" in the town.

It was not unusual for horses which had done little work throughout the week to be taken ill on the way into market from a disease known as *azoturia,* characterised now as haemoglobinuria, by a sudden and rapid swelling of certain muscles, usually those of the loins and quarters with extravasation of blood into their tissues. This was a very serious disease which frequently terminated in death or chronic wasting of the muscles.

Some of the horses affected with this disease would leave the farm perfectly well and go down in the road on the way into market, or get there and go down in the stable.

It was on one of these occasions that I was called to a stable in the town to attend an aged grey mare owned by a rather merry widow who kept a farm about seven miles from my surgery.

She was a large, stout but comely woman, who had visited the market for a number of years, always driving a very high trap loaded with baskets of butter, eggs and poultry, ready dressed, piled up in the back of the trap and on the seat alongside her own.

Her old grey mare had developed azoturia on the road into town but had finally managed to complete the journey. The widow had "sent for the vet," and started out on her delivery round on foot, with a basket on each arm. When I arrived at the hotel yard I found that the mare had gone down and was on the floor of the stable, sweating and struggling, surrounded by other horses. The police went out to look for the owner but could not locate her, and finally as the case was quite hopeless, I decided to destroy the mare and have her body carted away.

Madam must have had a good day's takings for she did not show up again, for as so often happened in her case, she fell in among friends and being a convivial soul, she indulged a little freely, and forgot all about the old grey mare.

She had not returned at 9 p.m. and the yard ostler was left to break the bad news to her when she returned. However, as it drew near closing time he, too, felt a need of refreshment and when nearly all of his farmer customers had returned home he retired to a nearby bar. While he was so occupied the widow returned.

I had to turn out to see an urgent case at 10 p.m. close to where the widow lived, and it was while I was returning home at about 11 p.m. in the light of the moon that I saw to my amazement, coming towards me, an apparition—the widow travelling at a great speed behind the grey mare.

I pulled up and got out of my car to investigate matters. As soon as the lady recognised me she let out a wild whoop of joy.

"Old mare's taken on a new lease of life," she shouted. "Whatever have you done to her? Never knew her trot along like this for last ten years."

"Where did you find her?" I asked.

"Took her from the stable myself. They'd moved her into a different stall, but I found her all right."

"How old was *your* grey mare?" I enquired.

"Twenty-two years come Michaelmas."

"Ah," I said. "That accounts for it., then. *This* one happens to be a four-year-old."

It was the most gentle way of breaking the news I could think of at the moment.

Every year, usually at half-way through March, or as soon as the likelihood of frost had gone, we would make arrangements to get busy castrating colts and calves, usually allotting one day or perhaps two in a week for the purpose.

This would include all the colts on the farms, bull calves and not infrequently a few adult bulls no longer required, and almost invariably the old boar pig.

There might also be a considerable number of colts among the wild moor ponies which would have to be operated on about this time of the year.

As a rule two of the firm went together on these expeditions since catching, roping, casting, tying and anaesthetising was a specialised task, and although roping and tying was hard work, it was a very personal matter when it was oneself that had to stand behind the animal tied up on the ground, and a foot suddenly becoming free could do one a serious injury. It was not a job that the average farm worker could be trusted to carry out.

Today colts are scarce, which is perhaps not such a bad thing from the veterinary angle when one remembers that horsemen are even more scarce, and it is almost impossible on a farm today to obtain help to handle the odd colt, since the only thing the average farm hand is capable of handling is a tractor.

Two of us, working as a team, could catch, cast, tie, anaesthetise and operate on as many as ten to twenty colts in a day, provided they were brought by their owners to one farm.

Since in Cornwall the animal population was so dense and farms were small, this often meant opening gates and driving colts together into one field. Very few of them, even as two-year-olds had ever been handled or haltered, so that a day's castrating was not only a surgical feat but it also bore many of the features of a rodeo without an audience, other than the farmhands, who were kept too busy to really enjoy themselves.

A great many of these colts were bred and raised on moors and hill farms, knew little about mankind and had decided objections to being haltered for the first time in their lives. As they used their fore and hind feet, and occasionally their teeth, as weapons of both defence and offence, and were particularly clever at standing up on their hind feet and boxing with their fore feet, the veterinary surgeon counted himself lucky every time he returned home unscathed at the end of the day.

As a rule we lassooed our colts, using a rope, the loop of which could only run up so far. A wooden peg spliced into the rope made it impossible for a colt to be throttled.

The colt was then driven into an open level field, four men running behind and holding the rope. Once in the middle of the field the men held their rope low to the ground and hung on to it with all their weight. Most colts would pull backwards upon them but occasionally we would encounter one which habitually galloped towards the men, instead of planting its feet and indulging in a tug of war.

As soon as the colt began to tire, it was *our* job to approach it. The rope which we used to cast and tie the colt was about forty feet long and made of cotton, which was soft and less likely to injure the animal's limbs. The two ends would be brought together and the centre tied to form a loop of suitable size which was to be passed over the head and neck, forming a circle around the neck, with two free ends.

The next performance was to get the loop around the colt's neck. This was done by first passing the rope held by the men through the loop. Taking one end of the rope each, the two people tying the colt, ourselves almost invariably, would slide the loop up the rope to the colt's head (not without remonstrance on the part of the colt) and endeavour to pass it over its head, often with the help of a long forked stick.

It must be remembered that to get within range of the colt's two fore feet would be almost equivalent to committing suicide, in the majority of cases.

When the rope loop had passed over the neck and the two free ends were held on either side of the colt, the next thing was to throw the ropes one at a time between the hind feet, and slipping behind the colt pick these up and keep them taut. One man would now hang tightly onto his rope (after the kicking match had subsided) while the other gathered up the slack in his, approached the colt's forehand and attempted to pass the end of his rope between the neckrope and the colt's shoulder. This was the most dangerous part of the procedure.

Your assistant on the other side of the colt, then passed the end of his rope also through the neckrope. The colt was held with these for a few moments until his resistance had diminished, each rope was slackened and allowed to drop over each hock into the heel of the foot.

When the men had been arranged, three or four on each rope, the signal to pull was given, the hind feet of the colt were drawn up to his elbows and he lay on the ground ready to be tied. This was another specialised job by which all four feet were securely lashed together by a somewhat complicated system of half-hitches.

I have described this procedure in detail not because many of my readers will ever have to catch, cast and tie a colt, but in order to make it plain that whoever repeated this procedure ten or twenty times in a day, in addition to having to get washed up and sterile in order to perform the operation, was no idler.

I doubt if very many of the public, people working behind desks or counters, have any idea of the strenuous work involved in a profession which necessitates constantly handling heavy animals. It will now become more evident why, earlier in this book, I advised every young man considering entering the profession to undergo medical examination before finally making up his mind which profession to select.

It is quite true that the castration of colts is carried out less frequently than of yore, even rarely in some practices, but when one type of work diminishes another takes its place and the handling of cattle can become quite strenuous on occasion.

Quite apart from the nature of the work the hours are long and exacting, and there is no guarantee of undisturbed rest, whenever the time for it falls due.

While writing about handling colts, I would mention that occasionally we came up against one with what might be regarded as possessing criminal tendencies.

I have in mind one Thoroughbred two-year-old which had already beaten two veterinary surgeons who had attempted to castrate it, inflicting injuries upon them both.

On our first attempt the colt kicked our assistant on the head and this postponed the operation for a week.

The second attempt was successful.

A year later, this colt after being broken to saddle, ran away with its new owner who was riding it, and jumped over the edge of a 300 foot cliff into the sea, drowning them both.

One of the most unpleasant tasks was the castration of the old boar, which having outlived his usefulness was to be fed to provide pork for the butcher.

Some of these had tusks, four inches in length, and were willing to use them on all and sundry.

One of my most unhappy recollections is of a large boar pig, which preparatory to anaesthesia had been tied by a rope applied around its upper jaw, behind the tusks, to an iron rail in a cowshed. The boar struggled, the rope broke, and the farmer, his pigman and myself, spent the greater part of the morning sitting among the beams beneath the roof while the boar sat below, champing his jaws and waiting for the first person to fall off the beams.

There we stayed until the farmer's son returned from market, saw what was happening, fetched his gun and shot the boar.

Before ceasing to discuss horse practice I would like to draw attention to a wartime picture, which we shall never again see. Whether we continue to have wars, one final cataclysm, or if we decide to live in peace, there will never again exist an army horse hospital of a large capacity.

During the First World War, after being rejected by nine medical boards on account of an alleged heart murmur which had never troubled me and has never done since, I applied to the Director of Army Veterinary Services at Aldershot to ascertain whether I might be employed in a private capacity. As a result I was sent as civil veterinary surgeon to a very large veterinary hospital in the south of England and put in charge of the department of surgery.

The hospital had accommodation for 4,500 horses and 1,000 mules, but most of the time it sheltered a far greater number.

The surgical ward had accommodation for 500 horses in boxes and stalls, and the whole hospital was staffed at the time of my arrival by 16 officers and 1,000 N.C.O.'s and men.

I had my surgical section to myself and as more and more officers were drafted for foreign service while I remained stationary, it became necessary for me to take over in addition to my own work the admissions, allot each animal its case card, and examine all fresh cases of lameness and make a tentative diagnosis before sending them to their own wards for treatment.

I was provided with two to three sergeants, several N.C.O.'s and plenty of men, but unfortunately, when interrogated, a great many of those sent to look after horses, appeared to have been in private life, actor-managers, jewellers, or drapers' assistants, or to have engaged in other occupations far removed from the care and feeding of horses.

We did get together, however, a little nucleus of hunt servants, and these were truly wonderful, and I shall always owe them a debt of gratitude. We used these men in the operating room and without them we should have been lost.

We had a great many imported and practically unbroken Canadian horses, and a large assortment of wicked mules, which were "wished upon" the surgical ward by those who had already had experience of their manners and habits. While I was at the hospital several of our men were killed by these mules. One man walking three feet in front of one of them, towing it along on a rope held over his shoulder, received a "cow kick" by which the toe of the mule's hind foot shot forward some distance in front of its ears, and completely removed the top half of the cranium of the man leading it.

The veterinary hospital was admirably laid out and fitted. It had an enormous operating theatre with two squads of men in attendance, seven in each squad with an N.C.O. and a sergeant-in-charge. All my patients were cast and anaesthetised ready for me to carry out the operation. While I was working at one end of the room, the next patient was being cast and anaesthetised at the other end. By this means I was able to perform from five to eight major operations a day, which was excellent experience for a young surgeon.

It was certainly non-stop surgery but it was made easy because every man knew what he had to do—and did it.

The arrangements in this hospital were a great credit to the late Lt. Col. A. S. Head, who was in charge at Headquarters.

We were enabled to carry out a good deal of research work in connection with operations then materialising for the relief of roaring, methods of cryptorchid castration, the surgical treatment of herniae and operations upon bone tissues.

Apart from the experience the young veterinary surgeons gained, much of which proved valuable to the profession subsequently, we were not entirely without amusement and we found most of this in equestrianism. We even ran one or two horse shows and built a small jumping course, which was helpful to those officers who had had little riding experience. It became part of my duty to issue remounts from the hospital, suitable for the officers concerned, and our riding school proved its usefulness.

What none of us realised was that most of the work we were doing and the methods of operation and treatment we were devising, so necessary at that time for maintaining our army and transport horses, would after another few years cease to possess much more than an academic interest.

Chapter Six

SMALL ANIMAL PRACTICE

THE TREATMENT of dogs, cats and other household pets, may be less exacting physically than large animal practice, but it is far more exhausting mentally.

The true animal lover, without indulging in rank anthropomorphism, possesses a rather sentimental type of mind and it does not matter in the least how long a veterinary surgeon has been in practice, he or she still grieves over the sufferings of sick patients, is sad when they depart this life in spite of all that can be done for them, and rejoices when they make good recoveries.

When I visit my veterinary friends, nowadays, I am always impressed by the fact that they worry about their cases and their patients. They develop an anxiety complex, so it is not at all surprising that both veterinary surgeons and doctors, constantly overworked, at the beck and call of clients at all hours of the day and night, worried, unconsciously maybe about their patients, become neurotic, often chain smokers, eat odd foods at odd hours—or little at all—develop duodenal ulcers and hypertension, and so frequently pass out in middle age from coronary thrombosis.

Not only are patients a source of anxiety but their owners, too, may provide even more worry than their pets.

Rightly or wrongly, a great many women pacify their own frustrations by bestowing their love upon animals.

Veterinary surgeons meet all kinds of people among their clients and must sometimes come to the firm conclusion that the owner is frequently in greater need of treatment than the pet.

Probably every practitioner is quite familiar with the type of woman who declares—as one did to me recently:

"Of course I've got Baby now, and I suppose that does make things a little better, but really, I think I'd feel losing my Peke just as much as losing the baby!"

This exaggerated affection for animals rather than for human companions is by no means a failing of the gentler sex. Strong men fall for their animals nearly as often as the ladies, as is evidenced by the following instance:—

The fond owner was a stout, middle-aged gentleman, a business tycoon, whose spaniel had fallen over a Cornish cliff, fracturing its shoulder.

When I arrived on the scene, the dog had been rescued and carried up to the cliff top by a perspiring coastguard with the aid of a long rope and some volunteer helpers.

The owner was sitting on the grass at the top of the cliff, weeping copiously and nursing the spaniel on his lap, surrounded by an interested and sympathetic crowd. At intervals he would dry his eyes and wail, "Oh! Why must it always be Bob? Why can't it be Sally sometimes?"

There was a stir in the crowd, and a charming little woman jumped out of a car which had just pulled up, rushed across the green and flung her arms around what proved to be her dog and her husband.

The gentleman, forgetting his grief for the moment, blazed out at her:

"For goodness sake, Sally, be a little more careful, will you? You'll hurt Bob's leg."

Every veterinary surgeon has encountered, too, the embarrassing female, usually middle-aged, whose Peke sleeps midway between the pillow and the foot of the bed, between the sheets.

This tiresome animal invariably chooses the small hours of the morning, or breakfast-in-bed time, to exhibit symptoms which throw its mistress into an uncontrollable flurry. The need for clinical examination of the patient always appears to necessitate its extraction from the most embarrassing locations. Once secured, it snarls, snaps and attempts to bite friends or acquaintances without fear or favour; then retreats strategically back to its original shelter beneath the bedclothes.

The owner is invariably one of those exacting persons who refuse to accept the services of an assistant, and the badly concealed joy in the faces of all the staff when the lady is on the 'phone awaiting attention, is to say the least about it, very depressing.

Then, one has to deal with those exasperating people who turn up at odd moments, quite outside surgery hours, and expect immediate attention.

One is probably already in the car, in the dickens of a hurry to keep an appointment, or late starting on a long round.

"So fortunate to catch you," they say. "We only want Bo-Bo's nails trimmed, and perhaps you wouldn't mind scaling his teeth and cleaning his ears." Then, as an afterthought: "We did take him to another veterinary surgeon last week, but he couldn't handle him like you do, so Bo-Bo bit him."

Politely you point to the notice on your surgery door which plainly states your hours of attendance. You apologise and ask to be excused as you have a pressing engagement.

"Oh dear!" says one lady to the other. "Whatever shall we do? I never realised that veterinary surgeons had real surgery hours. Almost like a proper doctor, isn't it, dear?"

When one realises that the average veterinary surgeon has to put in fifteen or sixteen country visits in a day, perform several operations, attend two hours or more at surgeries, carry out his Ministry of Agriculture work and Public Health service, examine a hunter perhaps, write his many reports and attend to a voluminous correspondence, all in the normal eighteen working hours, a careless remark such as the above from a casual owner can prove quite irritating unless one is endowed with a generous sense of humour.

A great many of the cases veterinary surgeons are called upon to treat in dogs, arise from their having swallowed a foreign body of some kind.

In days gone by dogs not infrequently swallowed the wooden skewer which impaled the separate pieces of "cat's meat." I have known large puppies, particularly Great Danes, swallow the dessertspoon out of which they were taking their daily dollops of cod-liver-oil. Fortunately these accidents are amenable to surgical treatment.

The most unpleasant articles dogs, and cats, swallow are needles. The needle is usually threaded. The animal plays with the thread, or wool, swallows it, and the needle follows.

In the summer, in holiday times, when Father fishes off the pier, using a herring bait, and knocks off for a smoke, his dog may swallow the herring. In his anxiety its owner tries to pull the line out of its mouth—and the damage is done. There were very few summers passed on the Cornish coast during which we were not called upon to remove fish hooks from dogs' interiors.

From the intestine of an Airedale, I extracted one half of a rubber bone, which the owner claimed to have destroyed. Six months later the dog came back again with the same trouble. Whether the second and the first halves were the same or made a pair, I never discovered. Unfortunately there is no law to prohibit the sale of rubber bones to innocent dog owners. They provide a lot of employment for veterinary surgeons.

Domestication has rendered our dogs liable also to many disorders which in a state of nature they would escape. Teeth are lost from pyorrhoea, engendered by soft food. Hearing that large bones are a useful preventive, owners forget the adjective "large," and give the dog the chop bones and the carcase of the chicken. More surgery is then required in many instances.

A good many dogs have a hankering after nylon stockings and swallow them whole. Their removal is made more difficult when the two stocking are present inside the dog, tied together at their feet.

The attempts of breeders to produce dogs to correspond with a standard which demands freakish development introduces genes which bring into the strain such eye diseases as cataract, prolapse of the lens, retinal atrophy and other conditions terminating in blindness. This sort of thing is encouraged also by those who go in for mass production of puppies (notably Poodles nowadays) for the pet market. Some breeds such as Dachshunds and Pekes, have now developed spines with a life of only four to five years. The result is paralysis due to "slipped" or "exploded" discs at this early age.

A common disease of dogs is nephritis, an inflammation of the kidneys which may attack from various causes at all ages, but is one of the common causes of death in dogs over middle age.

In younger dogs it may be contracted from lamp posts, the organism which carries it being eliminated in the urine of an affected dog, who may catch it in the first place from food contaminated by rat urine. Another very serious disease, leptospiral jaundice, is also spread by rats.

I need not say a great deal about canine distemper, its modern variation "hard pad," or any of the other virus diseases of dogs. They are terrible in their effects.

Fortunately all can be prevented by the vaccination of young puppies, with a second dose of vaccine at ten to twelve months. It would be criminal for anyone who owns a puppy and has any regard for its welfare, and a hatred of suffering, to neglect this elementary precaution.

In small animal diagnosis, nowadays, as in human medicine, the examination of blood and x-ray examination are routine practices, and when remote organs such as kidneys, bladder or spinal cord are involved, processes are made use of by which suitable dyes make the interiors of cavities resistant to x-rays and show up their defects.

From the viewpoint of both medicine and surgery, when we consider prevention, diagnosis or treatment by modern drugs, or by surgical intervention, there is nothing carried out in the human being which cannot be repeated in the animal body. Surgery, as carried out in animals, has made immense strides. Thirty years ago, it would not have been considered possible that certain forms of blindness in dogs could be overcome by grafting in the cornea from a healthy dog which had died. Nor would dogs suffering from cataract have their lenses extracted as a routine or everyday type of operation.

The surgery carried out by veterinary surgeons on animals is often of immense value to human surgeons who wish to determine whether certain delicate operations on the human body are likely to be successful.

The examination of urine, a routine practice in man and animals, is not quite so simple in one respect in animals as in man. This applies to its collection. The use of the catheter in animals is apt to produce misleading results, and most animals are more shy than human beings in the matter of their personal habits.

I remember attending a spaniel dog, the property of a dear little old lady, very Victorian in her ways, who lived entirely alone, except for her dog, in a Cornish market town.

I suspected that her pet was developing nephritis and I asked the lady one evening if she thought she might be able to collect a sample of his urine. She was quite sure she could do so and would have the sample ready for me on the following day at noon.

This happened to be market day when the streets were crowded with farmers and their wives, all agog to see the sights of town. This time they were not disappointed.

At midday when I drove into the town I could see by the queer way certain acquaintances grinned at me, that something was afoot. As soon as I got out of my car I was enlightened. A farmer came up to me and said:

"A brave joke we've been having this forenoon. A little old lady, in an old-fashioned bonnet has been running up and down the main street all the morning. She had a spaniel running alongside and she carried its lead in one hand and the baby's chamber in the other. Every time the dog stopped, she bent down and pushed the chamber under it. When the constable asked her why she was acting so queer, she told him *you* had told her to do it.

"She was successful at last outside Forster's butcher's shop. She had a crowd with her all the way, but *she* didn't worry!"

I got my sample all right and the dear old soul made no reference to any difficulty in collecting it—nor did I enquire.

Veterinary surgeons who carry on a good deal of small animal practice, and those who devote their whole time to it, have several kinds of clients to deal with. These are firstly the ordinary everyday people who keep a dog as a pet and become very fond of it, regarding it, in fact, as a member of the family.

Secondly, there are the less sentimental, more commercially-minded clients, who breed dogs, not always with an eye to show but to providing puppies for the pet market. These people do not always consider the best interests of the breeds they patronise, and a great deal of the hereditary disease which is fast creeping into British kennels (and in other countries, too), is due to breeding from inferior bitches mated sometimes to close relations, and at others to dogs with a low stud fee dependent upon the fact that they are not in demand by the people who breed dogs on more scientific lines with a view to producing better and better specimens.

I am not suggesting for a moment that successful breeding depends merely upon paying expensive stud fees, for a good many of the dogs which command high fees are sometimes quite undesirable as sires from the genetic standpoint. At the same time the really good dogs also command equivalent fees, and in dog breeding, as in most other pursuits, one seldom gets the best without paying for it.

The final category into which clients fall includes the bona-fide breeder-exhibitors who regard dog breeding as a hobby and a challenge, rather than as a way of making money. I think it is a fact that the majority of these desirable people actually put their hands into their pockets to pay for the pleasure they derive from their hobby.

The spirit of competition is very keen among breeders, which is as it should be, for without it half the joy would depart. Human nature being what it is, a little jealousy must creep in sometimes, but this breaks no bones, and it is accepted throughout the dog fancy that whenever a fellow breeder is ill, strikes a bad patch, or is really in difficulties, fellow breeders rally around and do their utmost to set him, or quite frequently her, on the level again. Breeders are like some families; they quarrel among themselves but stick together like glue when they are unjustly assailed.

Sometimes enthusiasm tends to run away with dog fanciers, as it does with those devoted to other pursuits.

I heard of a sad case recently which concerned a keen lady exhibitor, who really lived for her dogs.

By some means she found time to get married, and many of us who admired her, were keen to congratulate the happy pair. But we were a little surprised when she set off on her honeymoon with her bridegroom, who was not terribly keen on dogs, sitting on one side of the railway carriage, while the bride sat on the opposite seat with three cocker spaniels on her knees.

I heard later that when they booked in at their seaside hotel the rooms were quite small and the hotel was very crowded, so the bridegroom had to go elsewhere and book a single room for himself.

No veterinary surgeon can remain in practice very long without discovering that a great many dog owners, usually exhibitors, try to persuade him to carry out "beautifying" operations which may satisfy the aesthetic cravings of a show judge, but do little to benefit the dog, and may even cause it a certain amount of suffering.

The owner of a very tiny Pomeranian once caused me considerable embarrassment, in her efforts to persuade me to do something on these lines.

I should mention that the incident occurred a good many years ago before the invasion of immigrants from Jamaica, and it happened in a Cornish seaside town where sailors of all colours and nationalities were in the habit of calling.

She was a frowsy-looking woman and she walked unannounced into my surgery at a very inappropriate moment, while I was sounding the heartbeats of a Pekingese, and its lady owner was sitting in a chair watching me and awaiting my verdict very anxiously.

I noticed as I looked up, but without any particular interest, that the woman was carrying a small dog and dragging a child by the hand.

She stood behind a high table, resembling a shop counter in construction, and I could see only her upper portion and the Pom she carried tucked in her arm.

I suppose I glanced rather severely at her but she was not daunted. She burst out in speech, very hurriedly:

"Sorry to butt in, but I've a bus to catch, and only a few minutes to spare. I wanted to know when I can bring this bitch puppy in for you to touch up a bit."

I could see she was an impatient type of woman and had not the slightest intention of allowing me to attend my patient until I had answered her question.

"What is the trouble?" I asked. I could see there was no other way to be rid of her.

"Can't you see? The puppy's got a pink nose."

"Well, what about it?" I asked.

"I want you to DO something about it. Tattoo it or something. I want to show her at ——— in a few weeks' time. Never had a pink nose all the time I've been breeding."

She began to weep. An odour of gin pervaded the surgery.

"I don't see anything to make a fuss about," I replied. "There are worse troubles in the world than pink noses, I should imagine."

She wept some more.

"What trouble could a woman have," she wailed, "worse than a black Pom with a pink nose?"

"Well," I replied in desperation, rather foolishly perhaps, "I suppose she *could* have a black baby!"

Something seemed to have happened, quite suddenly. The whole atmosphere changed. She flashed at me a glance in which all the venom in her nature seemed to be concentrated. Then she wheeled round and dragged out her squalling infant by the arm. The child *was* black!

When primitive man and the wild dog first went into partnership, the arrangement was on a fifty-fifty basis. The man ate the food the animal caught or collected, and the dog got the leavings, if there were any. Probably nobody bothered a great deal about the other partner so long as it continued to deliver the goods. The little matter of affection had not yet begun to complicate the relationship, and in those days nobody had recognised the degree of uplift which the society of animals is supposed nowadays to confer on their human associates.

Puppies were probably plentiful. They made excellent bed-warmers for the children and when they became fat they were equally excellent, roasted over wood ashes.

Soon after this, when affairs got really tough, men began to notice that after all their friends had remembered engagements elsewhere it was only the dog that continued to hang around. But it took a good many centuries for this to sink in for man is at the best a selfish creature, especially as regards his women and other pets.

As a lover of dogs, I would give one piece of advice to all who have surplus puppies. Never *give* one away. If you are interested in the happiness of the dog make someone pay for it. If people do not value a dog sufficiently to do this they will certainly never spend money to feed it properly. If a man pays heavily for a dog he will take care of it, brag about it to his friends, and keep it in good condition.

I would not insist upon payment from most women, unless the lady in question had young children, when I would hesitate about letting her have a puppy at all, unless it was one of a large and powerful breed—in which case she would not want it.

Women are motherly creatures as a rule—there are exceptions—and therefore kinder to animals, but a few are exhibitionists and love dogs mainly for the notice men take of them.

You cannot fail to have observed the large stout lady who cuddles a miniature Peke to her ample bosom, or the diminutive young lady who delights in being hauled around the town by a massive Great Dane, or a graceful Borzoi. I knew one girl of four feet nothing, who kept an oversized golden retriever in a tiny flat "for protection."

Every time it wagged its tail it broke something, on one occasion a new tea set.

Dogs in these days are certainly needed in lonely places, more so perhaps in town than country. Unhappily, as a rule, it is the wrong person who gets bitten, which is unfortunate for the dog—it isn't always the best workman who gets the most cake.

All veterinary surgeons are only too familiar with the owner who condemns a dog to be "put to sleep" when it is not the dog that is at fault but the owner, who has taught it to guard the house without telling the dog, or making it understand, which people are friends and which are foes.

Too many pets are kept merely for the pleasure they afford the owner. So few owners give equal pleasure to their pets, forgetting that the environment and way of living which pleases an owner may not appeal to a four-legged pet in the slightest degree.

It is odd how the treatment afforded to various pets by their owners varies, even in different localities. Some dogs are over-pampered, become fat and irritable, while others are neglected and half-starved. A dog will forgive its master for starving it but will break its heart if it is neglected and goes unnoticed. Farm dogs are often frightfully neglected, tied beneath a cart, and have food, a crust of bread perhaps, thrown them when somebody remembers.

January is the month when the old dogs, as well as the puppies which have reached their six months exemption, are "taken to the vet" to be put to sleep, or are taken out in the car, dropped on a lonely road, and "lost." This latter method of getting rid of the dog is an offence I think should be punished by imprisonment.

The six-months puppy no longer amuses the baby and is not worth a licence, so it must be "bumped," according to the expression made use of by the class of people who put this procedure into practice.

One cannot work as a veterinary surgeon for long without discovering that a large proportion of humanity regards animal life as of no account whatever, and considers they are as justified in condemning a loyal and trusting canine pal to death as they are in swatting a bluebottle.

If one attempts to explain that the life of an animal is not to be taken lightly, and when one points out the time and trouble that is often given to *saving* life, the owner of the dog looks at one as though one were bereft of one's senses. The dog is his—or her's, as the case may be—it is only a dog, and it is unwanted. What can be more natural than to have it destroyed?

There is no answer to the client with this type of mentality. The only consolation is that the dog may be happier, dead, than compelled to live with a person temperamentally unfit to have charge of any kind of animal.

Veterinary surgeons know full well how greatly animal owners differ in the amount of attention they are willing to expend upon the welfare of their pets and also how much in hard cash they are willing to lay out for treatment to prevent illness, or to secure their recovery when ill.

It is quite common for a working man to pay several guineas for an operation on a pet of no intrinsic value, even when doing so means self-sacrifice, stinting his beer or tobacco. In such cases one gladly lets the client off lightly, or accepts payment at the client's convenience.

On the other hand, many owners, well able to pay, are very stingy; they ask all sorts of questions and invent countless excuses to avoid treatment or payment, and decide that "it isn't right to let him suffer," and order the dog's destruction.

But if one feels sorry for the patient and willing to waive the fee in order to save its life, the owner at once consents to having the treatment or operation, whichever it may be, and all the scruples about letting the dog suffer go by the board.

But in many cases euthanasia cannot be avoided, and one of these once brought me into near-conflict with the U.S.A. forces.

I have often wondered what impression a party of G.I.'s must have taken home with them concerning a country village in England, in which they were billeted during the Second World War.

It was near its termination, and on a summer evening one of my clients who kept a public house some miles out in the country rang to say that his Great Dane dog had developed hysteria and was scaring the whole neighbourhood. It had bitten my client and his son, too, and he thought it would be better to put it to sleep.

I packed my euthanasia kit and also a .410 in case of emergencies, and drove to the village.

When I arrived I found that the dog, a huge two-year-old, was suffering from hard-pad, a type of distemper, and this was complicated by encephalitis, which was making the dog savage and ready to attack anyone who came within reach.

As nobody would volunteer to assist me in giving him an injection, I asked the owner's permission to shoot him, and I put a full charge of shot into his brain at close range killing him instantaneously.

The question arose as to how best to dispose of the body. In the normal way we used to place the bodies of small dogs in a metal container in the boot of the car, take them to town and have them cremated, but this dog was the size of a small donkey. The owner's wife was very insistent that the dog should be buried on the outer portion of the tennis court and, as the owner was agreeable, I concurred wholeheartedly with his wife's suggestion.

But the following afternoon the wife rang again. Her husband's hand which had been bitten, as well as his arm, were badly swollen and he was unable to dig the grave, nor could he find anyone in the village who would take over the job. Could I possibly send someone to collect the body?

It happened that nobody on my staff was available, so rather than leave the carcase unburied another night, I decided to go myself.

I took the old Ford we kept for such odd purposes and we managed to lay the body on sacking on the floor of the back of the car and cover it with a tarpaulin.

I had travelled only two miles on the road back to town when I was "assailed" by a party of three G.I.'s who wanted a lift. I told them I had no available space but they pointed at the two empty back seats and began to get a little awkward. So I told them they could ride at their own risk, and in jumped the three, two on the seat and one stretched out at full length on the tarpaulin covering the body.

As we proceeded towards town I kept an eye on the party through my driving mirror. I could sense a gradually increasing uneasiness building up behind me.

Presently the gentleman reposing on the tarpaulin sprang up, and hanging on to the back of my seat, he shouted:

"Holy Creepers! What's under that tarp?"

"A corpse," I replied.

"Corpse!" The exclamation came from all three at one time. "What kind of a corpse?"

"It's the corpse of a Dane," I replied. "He got a bit troublesome down at the pub last night—so I shot him!"

I pulled up the car so nobody would get hurt in scrambling over the side. I never saw any vehicle unload so rapidly.

I had proceeded only a few hundred yards when I began to overhaul a second party of G.I's and they, too, attempted to thumb a lift.

I tried to wave them down but at that moment my friends from down the road hove into sight and began to shout and signal to the others.

I decided not to hang about so I stepped hard on the accelerator in case there was any misunderstanding.

I wonder what sort of story circulated around their camp later that night? Chicago had nothing on that village by the time the recital had gone round a few times.

This all came about through a mistake in identity and while we are on this subject, I might close this chapter with two other incidents arising from the same cause.

I sincerely hope that the two stories I am about to relate will not also lead to any misunderstanding.

The ethics of the veterinary profession forbid its members to assume any degree of unusual importance, or to connect themselves in any way with behaviour which might savour of personal advertisement.

I trust, therefore, that none of my readers will imagine that I lay claim to any of the powers ascribed to me by my clients in either of these particular instances, and I would even categorically deny that I ever possessed them.

One of my assistants had called the previous day at a house hidden away on the top of a Cornish cliff to see a dog.

The patient was an aged black retriever dog, the beloved pet of an eccentric, nerve-ridden, old lady.

The following morning, in response to a frantic call on the telephone for my personal attention (fortunately it was this particular assistant's day off) I hastened to the house and arriving, a little out of breath, I was met at the front door by my client who was indulging in bursts of noisy weeping and showing every indication of acute distress.

"Thank heaven you've come yourself," she wailed. "I think Dick's been dead an hour, but *please* go in and see him and do what you can for him!"

She escorted me to the door of the sitting room.

I looked across the room at the body. It was stretched out on an old-fashioned sofa and over its tail end the dog's head hung limply at the full reach of its neck, its tongue hanging out of its mouth. Apparently life had departed.

"Is he dead?" she wailed.

"Yes! Poor old Dick! I'm afraid he's gone!" I answered.

With this, she emitted a series of shrill screams and rushed to the sanctuary of her bedroom.

I entered the room, closed the door, and laid my hand on the "corpse."

Dick lifted his head an inch, viewed me suspiciously through one eye, recognised me, and started to beat his tail violently up and down on the sofa.

A few minutes later my client returned. *I* was then on the sofa and Dick was sitting on the floor between my knees, his head cradled in my hands.

"Oh!" she screamed, "You wonderful man! He lives again, he lives! Thank Heaven you came yourself. Nobody else in the world, but *you, could* have done that!"

I am glad to relate that Dick and his fond mistress both lived another two years and, curiously, both passed away on the same day.

But I did not attempt any further resurrections.

To close this chapter I will record the second incident, somewhat on the same lines as the first. It merely relates the receipt of a latter from a grateful client. The letter read:

Dear Mr. ———

I am very thankful to tell you my dog has now completely recovered from his serious illness. As usual in time of trouble, I placed my faith in Our Maker, and all came well. I shall continue to do this in the future with complete confidence. I trust, however, I may be permitted to call on you in a case of dire emergency.

Yours faithfully,

———————

Chapter Seven

VETERINARY OBSTETRICS

I FEEL THAT the subject of obstetrics deserves a chapter to itself since birth, with all its complications, formed the basis of a great deal of work the veterinary surgeon was called upon to deal with in practice in country districts forty or fifty years ago.

Animals still produce their young in the same curious fashion but of late years one seems to meet with fewer cases of dystocia, or when one does it seems to be the fashion to perform a Caesarian operation without making any attempt to deliver the foetus through the normal passage. Whether this represents progress is a matter which might be debated with advantage. What the effect will be upon the new graduates who adopt this method of delivery without developing experience of foetal manipulation is also an interesting point. One thing is certain, that half the interest derived from country practice, the acquirement of an art involving manual dexterity (an achievement which is rapidly disappearing in obstetrical and other directions) will be lost when it becomes the general rule to deliver the young by means of the knife, rather than by the hand.

The country veterinary surgeon of many years ago was required to be equally expert in foaling, calving, lambing, farrowing and whelping.

Whelping bitches was largely carried out by the use of forceps, snares and button hooks, and those who were expert and could use their fingers to advantage, were in great demand and their efforts were usually successful.

Caesarian operations in bitches are perhaps more justifiable today than in cattle, since bitches appear to retain their fertility even after one or more operations, while cattle are far less likely to become pregnant again after their calf has been delivered in this way.

Some breeds, notably Bostons, and to a lesser degree, Scottish terriers and Pekingese, are notoriously difficult whelpers and Caesarian birth is quite common in these varieties.

Fortunately, perhaps, mares seldom foal, nowadays, except in racing studs where their veterinary attendants retain their manipulative skill, for although a few Caesarians have been carried out successfully in mares, horses generally are not good subjects for abdominal surgical interference.

One of the studies which has received a great deal of attention during the past twenty years is the matter of infertility, particularly in cattle.

But even fifty years ago we were quite awake to the matter and were even then treating this matter of bovine infertility and doing all in our power to keep the bovine population at a high level, particularly so, later during the war years, when we were greatly in need of dairy products as well as beef.

Veterinary surgeons, today, are rather apt to believe that it was they, who first drew attention to the scourge of infertility, and discovered that cows do not invariably average a calf a year as every dairymaid considers they should.

We, of an older generation, were no less active in its treatment, but we were handicapped by the fact that cows were, in our time, expected to conceive regularly to natural service; that venereal diseases peculiar to cows were transmitted regularly by this means; and that these were directly responsible for a great deal of infertility.

Today the majority of cows are rendered pregnant with far less difficulty by artificial insemination, now universally adopted, and as a consequence a number of diseases have virtually been eliminated.

Artificial insemination is now being used in dog practice for shy breeders. A letter received by my friend Cmdr. Norman Hinton, who writes regularly for Our Dogs, serves to show that the dog fanciers are keenly alive to its possibilities:

"Dear Sir,

My brother's tenant, a farmer, tells me his calves are born without the intervention of a bull, by some new principle, the name of the stuff being 'A.I.'

I am sure my wee Susie would appreciate the delicacy of this treatment, but neither ———— nor ———— (two well-known firms of chemists) sell it, and I wonder whether you could advise me where I could obtain a small bottle. She is very tiny and devoted to me but *hates* other dogs."

I would like to tell you something about my own introduction to the art of bovine obstetrics.

One must remember that in Cornwall, where I practised for the first thirty-five years of my professional career, quite a number of farms were run entirely by women, often with other women helpers from outside, sometimes with the help of one or more daughters. Not uncommonly some of the small holdings were carried on by only the occupier, frequently a widow.

On the occasion to which I am about to refer I was just sixteen and having passed the entrance examination for the Royal Veterinary College in London, I had already left school, and preparatory to commencing my studies I was proudly ensconced in my father's surgery in order that I might "see practice." Being afflicted with an inborn shyness I had mixed with other children but little and my worldly knowledge was terribly scanty. Beyond being vaguely aware that chickens came out of eggs, I had given no thought to the mysteries of nature, and the Facts of Life were, until presently, a sealed book to me. I was to have them brought somewhat forcibly to my notice quite shortly, although mercifully, I was unaware of the fact. I was alone in the surgery. My father was out on his morning round and as usual in my days of inexperience I was trying to do several things at one and the same time. Firstly, I was endeavouring to play the National Anthem on my brand new mouth organ, and whenever I found myself out of breath I reverted to my ostensible occupation, the polishing of an assortment of large and fearsome-looking steel instruments, the use of which I neither knew or suspected.

On this particular morning I had all the instruments laid out for my father's inspection upon his return when there was a loud ring at the surgery bell and into the room marched one of the biggest and fattest women it has ever been my lot to behold. In her hand she carried a short, useful looking whip and she was clad in the fashion of country women of that day, in thick, black bodice and skirt, heavy wool stockings and a remarkably hefty pair of hobnailed boots.

"Where's your father?" she demanded.

In awe-stricken tones I managed to convey the information that I was alone and that my father might be absent some hours.

The lady appeared to be somewhat taken aback by this piece of information but she quickly rallied. Her eyes glued themselves on the array of instruments laid out upon the table and there came a gleam of triumph into her gaze which convinced me that there was much trouble in store. As events proved I was correct and there was very little doubt in my mind as to who was about to become involved in it. Her next remark settled it.

"You'll do," she said. Probably I looked a little blank. "Pack them up," she cried, pointing at the instruments: "the old cow's calving. I'll drive you out."

I made some feeble attempt at remonstrance but I was as wax in the hands of that dominant female. In mesmerised compliance I packed the instruments into my father's bag and had enough presence of mind to leave a note on the desk: "Gone to Mrs. Martin's, Constantine." Then, almost before I realised it, I was sitting on the spare seat of a high, dilapidated dog cart, behind an equally disreputable old grey mare, and we were on our way to my introduction to veterinary obstetrics.

Nobody can appreciate the agony I endured on that seven-mile drive. Conversation flagged. Madam was absorbed in her contemplation of the tragic fate which might even now be befalling her beloved "old cow." I was absorbed in contemplation of the fate which might presently overtake my father's unhappy pupil. We arrived.

It is an odd sight when first raw adolescence gazes upon the miracle of birth. I have thought many times since that Nature may have been a little thoughtless when designing the anatomical outlay of the female form but never was I more convinced than when my gaze first rested on Madam's old cow. Nothing less potent than a fire brigade could have washed away the filth which seemed to surround her from every angle. In the midst of this I espied a blood-stained infant foot—and was promptly sick.

Madam either disregarded this little incident or attributed it to natural causes, for her next instruction to me was to remove my jacket and shirt. Gingerly I took off my coat and waistcoat and commenced to roll up the sleeves of my shirt.

"That won't do," she cried. Off with that shirt and vest. Your father always does."

There was no help for it so I obeyed. My shame was terrible; I felt my cheeks burning but there was no escape.

I turned and looked upon my patient. As a child, the Hampton Court Maze had always greatly intrigued me; I had a picture of it in one of my school books. The Maze, according to the diagram, appeared to be simplicity itself compared with the impression I gathered of the layout of that bovine matron.

I could sense Madam's impatience. She could contain herself no longer. I heard a loud swish right beside me. I dared not look, I knew instinctively; the black Alpaca jacket! Hastily I turned and dived frantically into the realms of midwifery, the lesser evil. Another swish, this time softer. I dared not look behind me but once more I knew! Gladly would I have scrambled to join the calf but there was no room for us both.

From behind me I could feel Madam's arms pushing past my own, then worse. I was becoming engulfed; I was suffocating!

And then, at last, I heard a sound in the passage outside. The door flew open and my father was standing before me. I was saved!

The whole existence of the Cornish farmer and of all the inmates of his household was in my younger days linked up with the welfare of his dairy herd, and it will readily be understood that he was greatly dependent upon his veterinary surgeon who was at one time his counsellor, adviser and friend, and often over long periods his creditor. Conditions on the farms have now greatly improved but back in those days a sick cow was the concern not only of the owner but of the whole village. Neighbours would drop in at all times of the night and day with advice, little bits of fancy foods for the patient; herbs, elder tea and all sorts of cure-alls. All of this passed the day away very harmoniously until bedtime; by then the farmer had become worked up to such a pitch that he was convinced that the end of the cow was not far distant and at that hour everybody began to feel the same way about it and he would be persuaded by one and all to "send for the vet." This sort of thing invariably happened in my own practice when there was trouble with calving, and after one and sundry had "had a go" and declared themselves beaten the early hours of the morning would have arrived and I would be hurriedly fetched. It always appeared, too, that although the farmer had had a lot of company throughout the whole of the day, now was the moment for everybody to drift off home. It was the "vet's" job and no doubt he would attend to it. This might have betrayed a very gratifying degree of confidence but things did not always turn out just like that. A calf is not a seven pound infant but represents possibly a hundred pounds of solid flesh and bone, jammed into a very confined space, and it often requires the combined strength of two or three men to effect delivery under the expert guidance of the veterinary surgeon, and nine times out of ten those men would have discreetly vanished by the time of his arrival.

On such occasions one was usually greeted by some half-awake individual recruited from among the neighbours.

In cases when the farm was run by a widow, a common occurrence, the man called in at such times was usually very bad-tempered at being disturbed from his rest, and entirely without sympathy for the poor veterinary surgeon who "was supposed to do that sort of thing."

This disgruntled individual was provided usually with one hurricane lamp, the flame of which flickered fitfully through its glass, which was blackened by the smoke of ages.

In cases such as this, while your dismal helpmate was trying to find the soap and to heat some water on a decrepit stove, the jet of which seemed always to be choked at that essential moment, you commenced to strip to the waist, hang your clothing on any convenient nail you could discover and don an ice-cold rubber overall. By this time if your luck was in, your helpmate would have assembled a towel and a dish containing a small particle of soap, by now rapidly dissolving. The dish would be greasy as you would discover as the fat worked its way under your nails as you strove to recover the remains of the soap. When you made an examination of your patient you would invariably find some serious trouble which would require the help of at least another couple of men, so you would send your helper off to wake and gather together some of the neighbours. For the next half-hour while you are waiting and half-freezing you leaned against the barley tub and repeated softly and slowly over and over again, all the swear words your repertoire has accumulated ever since you left your mother's knee. Then you set to wondering at what hour you would get back to bed but soon you give this up too, because you were perfectly aware that there would be no more bed for you on this particular night and you preferred not to face up to all the facts at the moment.

Footsteps in the lane, one by one, with tedious intervals between the arrivals as the neighbours, about twice as many as you would require, foregathered. Some were melancholy, some plainly annoyed, but every one would be filled with an overpowering curiosity. Each wanted to find out what the new "vet" was like and wondered whether he would be able to take a rise out of him before his neighbours. Unfortunately there was a monotonous sameness about their conversation; after the second round one began to dread the arrival of the next man; this was an event in *their* lives but not in that of a country veterinary surgeon. From experience one could pretty well predict the next question that would be asked and the joke which would circulate presently among all those tough miners or farm workers pulled out from their beds. One felt very weary at such times, especially when some knowledgeable individual, who so far had not been very helpful, started to offer advice and a long account of all the difficult cases he had dealt with when he was foreman to Lord So and So. All this would prove exasperating but you dared not show it, so you decided, rather than fell him with an embryotome, to give him a rope to pull.

Everything seemed to go wrong on such occasions. Usually, the cow upset the only available drop of warm water and more had to be fetched and heated; bundles of straw had to be fetched from some remote part of the farm buildings; the ropes you were depending on for traction decided to break at critical moments, and you wasted weary minutes affixing others while you alternately sweated and shivered with cold, and your hands ached and your arms became chapped from continuous rinsing. Eventually, after several hours, most of which time you had been lying upon a wet and filthy cowshed floor, the job was finished, and you washed your sweating, bloodsmeared body in the thick, cold, soupy water which remained, got someone to dry your back on the sodden towel and commenced to put on your clothes. By this time your collar stud would have been trodden into the dung underfoot, your vest would have been knocked off the nail upon which you hung it and would probably be reposing in a pool of liquid manure, and eventually you set off homewards wearing your overcoat, probably with last week's News of the Universe next to your skin.

For all this effort you would be paid, some day perhaps, little more than the consulting surgeon charged to take a look at the baby's tonsils. This was no reflection upon your skill or usefulness but was based upon the commercial value of the patient. Presumably babies were worth more than cows, although every smallholder agreed that a cow was very hard to replace.

Some of my clients in the more out-of-the-way moorland farms, fifty years ago, were very primitive in their way of life. I remember going one evening to just such a farm to foal a mare. When I arrived I was greeted by a woman who was evidently the boss, as in the dark background hovered a nondescript little man and five children of descending ages. Mentally I noted their seeming swarthiness and soon I was to guess the reason. When I asked the woman to procure me warm water, some soap and a towel, I observed her expression of dismay.

"You can have a "wiper," she said, "and some water, though not hot, seeing the fire's out this time of night, but you can't have any soap."

"And why is that?" I asked.

"Well, I did belong to keep a piece of soap, but six weeks back the woman uplong the next farm, 'er sent down and borrowed it. I've been meaning to ask for 'un back, but a week or two after 'er'd 'ad 'un, 'er sent down 'er little maid with twopence, so I 'avn't 'ad none since!"

Talking about lack of help reminds me of another farm, owned and worked entirely by a young and buxom widow in a rather out-of-the-way place, not far from Truro. I was called out on a Saturday night early in the evening and found only the widow there to help me. She explained that on that night of the week everybody had gone by 'bus or by train into Truro and there would be no help available. We did the best we could but were not making much headway, when I heard a man running along the road. I dashed out after him and he explained to me that he hailed from Redruth and was late for his train at the local station a mile along the road.

Well, I struck a bargain with him. He would stay and help me, and afterwards I would drive him home. Everything went well but just as I was ready to leave, a farmer rode in on a motor cycle from a farm about five miles further on. He had a horse very ill and on ringing my surgery had been advised to try to catch me before I left. I explained the situation and the widow kindly suggested that my helper should stay and have a wash and a dish of tea and that I should pick him up on my way back.

On the following Monday morning I thought as I was in the district I would call and see how my patient was progressing and I had turned into the yard before the terrible thought struck me. I had completely forgotten all about the man I had left there on the Saturday night! The widow came out to me, all smiles.

"Where the dickens is that man?" I asked.

"Oh! He's all right. Hasn't come down from bed yet."

Presently the gentleman appeared, not at all angry apparently.

"'T'es all right," he said. "We Cornish don' take no offence over the likes of a little thing like that. You shall take me home and go in first and explain it all to my missus."

I could see no help for it, so I did as he suggested.

I daresay he was quite right about Cornish people being pretty broadminded but there was one thing he forgot to mention. My friend was a Cornishman, but the moment she opened the door I saw—and heard—my error.

His wife hailed from Aberdeen!

That next half hour was one best erased from memory.

I mentioned earlier that at the time I first set up in practice on my own account, a number of unqualified persons were employed by farmers to attend cows experiencing difficulty in labour.

The custom became less and less common as the years rolled on and at the present time veterinary practice by unqualified persons, excepting in a few special circumstances, is illegal in Britain.

Nevertheless, some of these unqualified practitioners were remarkably efficient obstetricians, and the majority of them were well advanced in years. There were a few of the lesser lights, younger men, who were rough and clumsy, and depended on brute force rather than on manual dexterity, but these were in the minority.

The best and older men seldom encountered a case of dystocia they could not overcome by manipulation and traction, and I have known them succeed in producing live calves (and maintaining live mothers) in some of the most difficult cases, with very extraordinary presentations.

They scorned Caesarian section, which of course lay outside their range of activity, and although we were carrying out successful Caesarian operations in cases of foetal deformity as early as 1915, a great many equally successful operations had been recorded by other practitioners long before then.

But although the Cornish practitioners were able to operate quite successfully, most of them would have agreed completely with the unqualified men who specialised in calving cows, that it was only on very rare occasions that one met with the kind of foetal deformity or malpresentation which could not be dealt with successfully by manipulation.

When epidural anaesthesia came into use and it was possible after injecting a little of the anaesthetic solution into the root of the cow's tail, to effect delivery without the cow, which was otherwise completely conscious, continuing to strain or feeling any pain whatever, the few remaining local calving experts who were unable to adopt this procedure rapidly went out of business.

Farmers, for ever afterwards, called in their own qualified veterinary surgeons to all cows in which calving was not proceeding on normal lines. They soon found that Caesarian operations were rarely made use of by experienced veterinary surgeons, that their patients made rapid recoveries and owners experienced no difficulty in getting them into calf again, which they invariably did after a Caesarian operation.

I have vivid recollections of performing a Caesarian operation on a Guernsey cow during the second year of the last World War, when farm work was carried out mainly by Land Army women and German prisoners.

In this case the calf was not only oversize but it was markedly deformed, completely inside out, with all four limbs coming off from one portion of the body of the calf; one of the rare instances when Caesarian operation would be safer than embryotomy.

When I arrived at the farm prepared to operate, I found that the owner had decided to go away for the week-end and the only help available was supplied by one landgirl and one German prisoner. Before commencing the operation I explained quite briefly the kind of help I should want from each of them, and I think the landgirl took it all in, but as the German knew little English I doubt if he knew even what I was about to do. I could only hope for the best.

We succeeded in casting and tying the legs of the cow and administering the anaesthetic.

I had previously made my two helpers scrub their hands and arms and don two surgical overalls I had brought with me.

The landgirl was a well-built, buxom lass and fairly tall. I asked her if she thought she could stand seeing the operation without fainting in the middle of it, and she assured me she could. I refrained from asking the German since I could not speak German very fluently, and although he was not so big as the landgirl, he looked a regular cut-throat type who would have no "nerves," and might delight in bloodshed.

I had just reached that critical period when the calf had to be withdrawn through the flank incision. The landgirl was helping me and doing a first-class job.

We had the calf half-way out when we both heard a loud groan, and, glancing round, saw the German stretched out on the ground in a faint. We were working in a meadow adjoining a dense wood.

I said, "Leave him there a minute until we get this calf out."

But the girl was not listening. Screaming out, "Carl; Oh, Carl!" she ran over to the German, leaving me in charge of the calf, stooped down, lifted him up like a sack of corn, threw his unconscious form over her shoulder and staggered away with it into the woods.

I finished the operation alone, and I have never seen either of the pair since.

A week later I called at the farm and found it deserted, so far as humanity was concerned.

I found my patient out in a field feeding happily among a dozen other cows, so I returned home—still short of two sets of surgical overalls.

I once encountered a case in which the cow did not calve in a messy cowshed, or in the middle of a field on a wet night. One cow actually calved in the kitchen.

It was one of those old-fashioned farmhouses in which the house and out-buildings were continuous, and all beneath the same roof. By a little alteration the farmer had arranged matters so that the calving box was built onto the lower end of the kitchen, and by pulling back a sliding door the two compartments became continuous.

"I believe in a bit of comfort," the owner explained to me. "Home, here, I can sit in my armchair, smoke my pipe and watch the old cow calve. That's a lot better than getting in and out of bed."

He was right too. He kept a bottle of rum open on the kitchen table, and a saucepan half full of hot milk on the side of the hob. There are right ways and wrong ways of doing most things.

This calls to mind another true story related to me by Cmdr. Norman Hinton.

A cow was in trouble on a very bleak Gloucestershire hillside, on a bitterly cold winter's night. A dead calf had come away followed by most of the cow's internal organs. While the farmer stayed by her head, the veterinary surgeon, stripped to the waist and working by the light of a hurricane lamp, was carefully replacing the prolapsed parts. The job took nearly an hour, and when he had finished the veterinary surgeon straightened his back thankfully, and walked to the head of the cow.

"Why! She's dead!" he said to the farmer.

"Oh, aye," the latter agreed. "'er doid foive minutes arter you started. Oi wunnered w'ether oi did ought 'a tell 'ee, sir, but oi reckoned oi'd better not interrupt 'ee!"

One of my experiences associated with calving a cow was exciting while it lasted but had a tragic ending.

I was called in on a Sunday morning to attend a Guernsey cow which was held up in her calving.

When I reached the farm, which lay on the outskirts of a mining area, I was greeted by the lady of the house who had hot water, soap and towels in readiness.

She explained to me with many apologies that her husband was in bed, not at all well, and she feared I would have to manage without help. I thought this a little strange as on a Sunday, particularly, there was seldom any lack of neighbours in such circumstances.

The case was not at all difficult and everything was going nicely when a tousle-haired man, who apparently had overlooked his shaving for several weeks, wearing a dressing gown over pyjamas, rushed into the cowshed and commenced to abuse me quite savagely.

He declared I had come to kill his cow, and after a few more uncomplimentary remarks he picked up a shovel and commenced to take swings at my head, evidently intending to kill me.

I saw some implements stacked up in a corner of the shed and diving beneath the cow and coming out on her other side, I managed to grab a Cornish "eevil." I spell this word phonetically since I have never seen it in print, but it was a four-pronged fork, used for loading manure, with a five foot handle. This was the very weapon. I found I could keep the prongs close beneath the chin of my new acquaintance, while the handle of his shovel was too short to allow it to scalp me.

Evidently this dawned on my adversary, too, for suddenly throwing the shovel away he turned tail and marched out of the shed, across the yard and through a gate into a field.

I hoped he had not gone to fetch his gun, but as he did not return in a few minutes I completed the delivery of the calf, washed, got into my car and drove home to lunch.

An hour after my return the 'phone rang. At the other end was the local constable, speaking from the farm where I had calved the cow.

He told me that with the help of some neighbours he had recovered the body of the deceased, my acquaintance of the morning, from a disused mine-shaft situated in a field adjoining the farmyard.

Between the first and second world wars I engaged a young man, who was nineteen when he first came into my employment, to drive me and assist in holding animals on the farms.

Daniel was a keen exponent of Cornish wrestling and hanging onto the nose and horns of a wild steer appeared to be his particular form of enjoyment. In more ways than one, Daniel, loyal to the core, proved to be a pillar of strength, and I was very upset when the second war took him from me to show his prowess on a minesweeper rather than on the farm.

Daniel was very fond of driving a car and although he had enjoyed little schooling, he was very intelligent, and amused me greatly with his ingenuous outlook. What was equally gratifying was that he was always ready to turn out, whether by night or by day.

I used to keep my obstetric kit packed in a large, black wooden chest, a good deal like a coffin. It had a handle grip fitted at either end so that two people could carry it but Daniel always refused to let me help and would heave the chest onto his shoulder and carry it up the steepest hill.

I remember going with him one winter morning, about 5 a.m., to calve a cow on a lonely hillside farm.

The tracks leading to the summit were sheets of ice and of great steepness. We abandoned the car at the foot of the hill and began to climb in the darkness. Daniel, loaded with nearly half-a-hundredweight of ironmongery in the black chest, uttered never a word until we reached level ground at the top of the hill.

He lowered the box to the ground, pulled out his handkerchief and wiped his brow.

"I'll be darned, boss," he said, "if I can see what people want to go to Africa for—to climb the bleedin' Alps!"

I will conclude this chapter with a more pathetic story.

It was late at night, and tired after a long day's work I was just getting into bed. Then the 'phone rang. The message was from a young farmer, a man in the early thirties, with a dairy farm about five miles from my house. He had employed me on a number of occasions previously, but he struck me always as a shy, awkward type of man, one it was difficult to know at all well.

"I wish you'd come out as quickly as you can," he shouted through the earpiece. "I've got a bit of trouble on here and I'd appreciate your help."

"What is wrong?" I asked. "Another calving case?"

"Well, it's something of that kind," was the reply.

"I'll be right over."

I dressed again hastily, packed my black box into the car and was at the farm in about a quarter of an hour. As I approached the farm entrance the house was well lit up, and I could see my young client pacing up and down the road outside the gate.

By the light of my headlamps as I drew the car to a standstill, I could see, too, that his face was drawn and pale, and a cold sweat shone upon his forehead.

"Thank God, you've come," he said as I alighted from the car.

With that he seized me by the arm and propelled me, not into the yard but straight up the garden path, and up the steps to the front door.

I guessed that he wanted to pour out his troubles indoors before we went to the cowshed, but it soon became apparent that was not our destination.

Without checking his pace he half-led, half-pushed me up the stairs.

At the top was a bedroom door, slightly ajar and a light was showing through the crack.

He knocked on this, opened it very quietly and pushed me in, a little more gently than during our passage up the stairs.

Lying, half propped up in the bed, was his young wife.

"It's Mary," he said to me.

"She's due right now for her first, and she's awful scared-like. Ever since she saw you take that calf from the old Jersey a month back, she's had a terrible lot of faith in you. We thought, perhaps, you wouldn't mind dropping in like, and talking with her a little while."

He blushed all over his face, then shot out through the door, closed it behind him and left me alone with Mary.

I sat down beside the bed and took her hand in mine.

For the next half hour I talked to her softly and soothingly about the kindly provisions of Nature, how everything always adjusted itself, and there was no need for her to be afraid any longer.

When I left her she was in complete control of herself and quite confident that no danger threatened her or her child.

An hour after I had fallen asleep the 'phone by my bedside rang again.

"I thought I'd tell you," the voice came through, "everything's all right now. The pains started as soon as you left, quite rapid—like. Doctor's upstairs now and he says everything is fine. That was a wonderful job you did to Mary. We'll never forget it."

They didn't either. They called the baby after me; why, I can never imagine.

Chapter Eight

THE DIFFICULTY OF BEING A VETERINARY SURGEON

During my many years in veterinary practice I have often heard farmers remark that, in their opinion, it was far easier to attain success as a doctor than as a veterinary surgeon.

Although professional ethics never permitted me to agree or disagree, I must confess that, inwardly, I sometimes felt rather inclined to agree.

Of course, all that was back in the bad old days. Now in times when according to authoritative statement, "we have never had it so good," it might be even more difficult to say if the farmers who made the remarks quoted above, were right or wrong in their beliefs.

The doctor of today, through no fault of his own, has ceased in many instances to retain his place as the family counsellor to whom one confided one's troubles. In the old days he was a second father to every young person, and by the real fathers he was regarded as something midway between a family physician and a father confessor.

Nowadays, run off his feet by panel patients often suffering from imaginary or frivolous complaints, he spends a large portion of each day writing, filling up official forms, prescriptions and letters to the specialists to whom he donates his patients.

His surgery has become a sorting office from which the various types of illness are packed off to appropriate departments.

His patients become as sheep in the flocks gathered for hours, sometimes, in hospital waiting rooms, from which as out-patients they are sent to be x-rayed, subjected to various types of physical examination, chivvied by nurses and attendants, then returned to their doctor, or sent home to wait for months, maybe, before being dispatched to the operating table.

I refuse to believe that any self-respecting doctor of the old school, dedicated to his professional work, will ever admit that under the new regime he is happier, more proficient, more valuable, or more esteemed, than he was under the old system, in which he retained his independence.

The question of whether the doctor of today is to be regarded as successful or otherwise, hardly enters the question. Under the National Health Service he is just one cog in a complicated machine. His individuality has ceased to count.

Up to now the veterinary surgeon retains not only his individuality, but also, so far as any human being can do, he is able to exercise free-will. He sinks or swims, not through his proficiency or stupidity in the matter of filling up official forms, but according to whether he gives satisfaction to his clients and affords relief to his patients.

There is an ever-growing curiosity in certain sections of the profession, as to how veterinary surgeons might fare under a programme of national service, whether they would earn more, work fewer hours, whether they would specialise more, and if life would be happier or more miserable.

It is not for me to offer an opinion on such a matter as this, but many of our profession who for many years have been in close touch with medical practitioners, are fully cognisant of the risk one runs of being drawn into a situation in which one throws one's individuality aside, and becomes a small cog in a vast machine.

Leaving out, in either profession, the many occasions on which difficult situations can be smoothed out by an understanding of human and animal psychology, with perhaps the aid of a little legitimate showmanship, the diagnosis of a great many of the conditions encountered in man and in animals, demands an alertness and an ability to observe small details, which would put Sherlock Holmes, outside his consulting room, to shame.

But human patients can do what animals cannot do. They can talk, but whether the information they vouchsafe in this manner is better calculated to help their doctor, or confuse him, is another matter.

However, experienced doctors and experienced veterinary surgeons seldom have much difficulty in sorting the wheat from the chaff. The doctor may acquire information by way of his ears, which the veterinary surgeon also does, aided by all his other senses, especially the tactile impressions he receives through his finger tips.

This diagnostic ability to discover what goes on inside the body of a dumb animal is acquired more readily by those fortunate enough to be what is known as "animal-minded."

This does not imply that their skill and their ability to diagnose, is based on a greater degree of learning, but that the mentality of this fortunate human being is attuned to that of the animal. This is a quality which enables its possessor to "see" further than other people into the animal mind, sympathise with its outlook on life, and sense the conditions under which the animal lives.

So far as learning counts, the present young graduate is a long way in advance of the graduate of even twenty or thirty years ago. But, whether my age is playing tricks with me, or whether experience of life brings greater discernment I cannot say, but I feel sometimes that modern youth is apt to regard animals, other than man, as though they were the inhabitants of some world other than ours, and not as living, feeling creatures, with flesh and blood like our own, and subjected to the same joys, disappointments, discomforts and inconveniences which humanity shares with them.

To handle animals and live among them successfully, it is necessary to have an instinctive liking for them and to be able to sympathise with them in their griefs. A pretence of affectionate interest, even when supported by appropriate patter, deceives neither the animal nor the onlooker.

An elderly veterinary surgeon, who for a number of years shared with me the task of examining veterinary students, once exclaimed to me in a moment of exasperation:

"These lads today could blind their fathers with science, but they still cannot visualize an animal."

I think he meant to imply that while they could interpret visible signs of ill-health, they still failed to see the animal as a whole, as a living being in its artificial surroundings, mainly because the student's own background, upbringing and environment was completely different from that with which the speaker had been familiar in *his* youth.

This is a difficulty encountered by every modern veterinary student through no fault of his own. It is a fact that these remarks apply more particularly to male students. The women students have far greater perception and, of course, a great many of them have had far more experience of animals and have lived more closely in touch with them. Many girls ride ponies and horses, take an interest in equestrian sports and gymkhanas. They frequently breed and show dogs, while as children they kept pets.

Do the lads not do the same things? Very seldom.

They prefer motor cycles and cars to horses, they regard equestrianism as a pursuit suitable mainly for women; their interests lie in speed and space. And yet they choose animals as a means of livelihood!

This is the reason, undoubtedly, why women students usually outshine the men, and why women veterinary surgeons are to be found in the highest places, and in important posts on our University teaching staffs.

The older generations of veterinary surgeons were brought up from their youth to ride. Their only alternative would have been to walk.

Probably they hunted and found their enjoyment out-of-doors, usually in close companionship with animals.

But times have changed. The internal combustion engine has largely brought this about.

Cities and towns have crept out into the country. Horses and cattle have moved outwards, and now that so many people live in council houses and Corporation flats no dogs are permitted to be kept. Children have grown up among human beings, and riding, shooting, fishing, and hunting mean nothing to them. There are no animals in the cinemas and theatres, and horses in motion during racing and jumping may appear on television but do not attract young people to watch them.

None of this is written in any carping spirit or in any derogatory sense. It is something youth cannot avoid, one of the features of our new way of life. It would be impossible, we may suppose, for the youthful background and outlook to be other today than it is.

I am a little uncertain what the word "successful" really means in regard to the practising professions under present day conditions.

Success in the healing art should bear no relationship to pecuniary reward. Years ago our fees were small. Today, in keeping with modern trends and the present economic situation, fees are comparatively high, but whether practitioners enjoying greater comfort, and higher incomes are happier than we older people were in days long past, is still debatable.

A human patient tells the doctor in which limb he experiences pain, how it happened in the case of an injury, and he offers no active resistance to examination apart from a few grunts and groans when the part is handled. But when examining a dog or a horse, one has to determine for oneself which is the lame member—not always easy—and then find out which portion of the limb is affected and finally decide what is the pathological or surgical condition responsible for the pain or lameness.

The behaviour of an animal may suggest to the untrained observer that it is suffering from internal pain, but only the experienced clinician will be able to say definitely in what portion of the animal's anatomy the pain is located.

But the untrained observer is often led into error. Every veterinary surgeon is only too familiar with the anxious, agitated lady, who hastens to him with her young female cat which "has been rolling on the ground in "agony," and in *such* funny positions," when all the time this is the natural behaviour of young female cats during their period of oestrus.

Moreover, the inclination of the animal patient is to give no help, since it does not regard examination and treatment as something which is being done for its benefit and relief, but rather as an unwarrantable interference at a singularly inappropriate moment. So, instead of saying, "This is the leg that hurts. Please make it better," the average cow, for example, holds the aching limb carefully out of the way and makes a determined attempt to kick you as hard as possible with the sound one.

Then again, if one is to make or maintain a practice—and a reputation—and so continue to exist, surgical and obstetrical work has often, perforce, to be carried out with every appearance of success under conditions which would shock the surgeon who deals only with human bodies.

Nor is it correct to suppose that this sort of thing doesn't matter, or that animals have a far greater resistance to infection than mankind, or that they will survive an accidental infection which would kill off the average human patient.

The truth is that although surgical asepsis is always to be the aim, the human peritoneum is capable of withstanding far more interference than that of the horse or dog. The cow possesses rather greater peritoneal resistance and the pig one very much higher than any of these animals. Although the dog is liable to succumb to a comparatively slight infection of the abdomen, for some strange reason the cat appears relatively resistant to peritoneal infection but surprisingly prone to skin infection, and will develop an abscess, run a temperature and frequently die, from a bite from another cat, while a dog may be torn nearly in pieces by another dog, so far as its skin is concerned, and heal without any evidence of toxaemia or purulent infection.

As an instance of bowel contamination in a cat I have vivid recollection of a female cat which underwent ovaro-hysterectomy. After its return home, it sat in the kitchen, unchecked by its owner, licking the site of the healed incision the whole of the day, until eventually its intestines prolapsed. It then went out into the garden, dug a hole in the loose soil and buried its own intestines. The resulting telephone message stated that the cat was standing in the middle of the garden and seemed unable to move!

The intestines, fortunately intact, were dug up from the ground and washed with quantities of warm normal saline. They were replaced, and the wound was resutured in the usual manner. The cat never missed a meal and was walking about the following day as if nothing had happened. It made an uneventful recovery.

This was before the days of antibiotics, otherwise they would have obtained the credit for the cat's recovery.

But the least infection conveyed to the peritoneal cavity of a horse or dog, or even of a sheep, would result in death.

Until recent years abdominal surgery in the horse has been impossible, but nowadays flank incisions are used in cryptorchid operations, and for some types of surgery involving only the small intestine. The large intestine of the horse owing to its immense weight, the folding over of the colon and the size and position of the caecum, renders it impossible to carry out any operation upon it other than paracentesis, tapping the bowel with a fine trochar for the relief of tympany.

The cow is amenable to Caesarian surgery and to operations on the various stomachs and intestine, with a greater margin of safety even than in the human subject. I remember a resection of eighteen inches of the small intestine of a cow, carried out in a shed where cobwebs descended from the beams nearly to the ground, which was covered by a foot of manure.

A storm was raging outside and the animal was lying in the manure, refusing to rise and suffering from intussusception, a telescoping of the bowel.

A miniature tent made out of a boiled sheet was stretched over her. She survived the operation.

I wonder what a human surgeon would say if he were compelled to perform a similar operation upon a human being in such circumstances?

But all our abdominal operations do not go off quite so well under field conditions. Sometimes Fate is against one from the start, as it was in the case of the newborn Guernsey calf which was owned by two maiden ladies, who called us in to attend it.

The story was that it was born with its intestines hanging through its umbilical orifice. When I first saw the calf it was standing in a dirty cowshed with its intestines beneath its feet.

I told the ladies the case was hopeless but they insisted that something be done, and, very much against my better judgement, I anaesthetised the calf, opened up the abdomen, cleaned and replaced the intestines and sutured the abdominal wound. The calf came round from the anesthetic and appeared perfectly normal. I still gave a very dubious prognosis, and I was just getting into my car when one of the ladies said: "Oh! I've forgotten something."

She ran into the house and returned at once with a pudding basis containing a suspicious looking grey content.

"I put this," she said, "on the kitchen hob to keep warm. Did you need it?"

The calf did! It was its fourth stomach!

Stripping to the skin in a cold cowshed in the depth of winter was always an ordeal, in spite of much practice. Nor was it always easy to obtain warm water and soap in a country cottage in years gone by, especially when one was entirely dependent upon a wood fire and a large iron kettle.

But in the more civilised parts of Cornwall there were more amenities.

The eldest unmarried daughter, who might be sixteen or nearer sixty, had certain privileges or responsibilities, whichever way you choose to consider them, and she always took full advantage of the fact.

For instance, after a prolonged calving case on some of the bigger and better farms, I would be invited to bath before dressing myself for the homeward journey, or the next calving case.

I would be escorted into the parlour and there, in the centre of the floor, I would find a round bath, just large enough to sit down in, containing possibly four inches of tepid water.

Having completely disrobed, I would be required to seat myself in the bath while the eldest daughter sponged and dried my back, and Father and Mother stood looking on and giving general instructions.

I have even endured occasions on which the whole family would group themselves in chairs around the bath, and would watch me dress. On one of these, an old lady who was addressed by the young children as "Great-grandma," carried out a running commentary on the nature and quality of my undergarments, and even quoted the makers and the retail price of each article as I stepped into it.

But one can get used to anything, and country practice, all those years ago, was no exception.

To digress a little, it was another duty of the eldest daughter to warm the bed at night for visitors, as hot water bottles appeared to provide insuperable difficulties.

A greatly revered bishop once told me that on one occasion

when visiting one of his more remote Westcountry parishes, he was completely held up by the sudden descent of a moorland fog.

However, he was satisfactorily dined and wined, and on retiring to his room to rest he was amazed to find a plump and becoming maiden fast asleep in his bed. He wisely decided it might be better to descend the stairs to inquire whether the intrusion was an oversight or part of the customary courtesy.

When he reached the living room, he found it empty, all the family having retired to their rooms, and on returning to his bedroom he found that the maiden had awakened and flitted.

"However," the Bishop remarked to me, "she had fulfilled her social function—the bed was delightfully warm."

Keeping patients in hospital was always a worrying business, especially when for a great part of the time the dogs had to be in charge of kennel staff. Horses never escaped from boxes but dogs had a tendency to do so on the least provocation. I suppose I can consider myself lucky that only two dogs played this trick on me in fifty two years, and one of these was never officially admitted into the kennels.

The first dog I lost was an Airedale in my early days in practice.

I was living on the outskirts of a country town at the time, and the dog slipped its collar and ran away from one of my kennel lads whilst being taken for a country walk.

When I was notified, the lad and myself tracked the dog across fields, and were horrified to see him jump a low wall and disappear down a long disused mine shaft, which at that time were dotted about all over this part of the country.

Cautiously, we leaned over and looked down. There, to our surprise, was the dog only about twenty feet down, standing on a sollar, a stout piece of timber stretched across the mouth of the shaft. Below him there was a drop of probably two hundred feet before coming to water level.

The kennel lad raced back home and returned with his partner and a long coil of rope. As they were both convinced I was the lightest member of the party, I was chosen by mutual consent to make the rescue. The rope was tied below my armpits encircling my chest. I climbed over the low wall and down I went. The dog seemed delighted to see me, it had done all the mining it cared for by now. Sitting astride the sollar, which seemed a little frail and rotten, I took the rope off my shoulders and lashed it around the dog as well as I could. The boys heaved away and up he went. So far, so good.

I was considerably relieved when I saw the rope again descending.

I fixed it firmly around me and signalled the lads to pull.

But nothing happened. The rope jerked, gave me a nasty jab in the solar plexus, and that was all. Apparently one lad still had to hold the dog and they were unable to lift me. So there I remained for another hour-and-a-half until they arrived back with two labourers.

It was not my happiest hour and a half though I consoled myself with the thought that if the sollar collapsed beneath me the rope would still hold me. It was only after I had again reached terra firma that the lads confessed that before rusing off for help they had forgotten to make fast their end of the rope!

The second case concerned an oversized Sealyham. It seems that the owner called and dumped the dog in my kennels with a message that he would 'phone me after lunch.

Unfortunately, before he did so, I went to the kennel, thinking it was unoccupied, opened the door to admit a dog I had with me—and away went the Sealyham.

It transpired later that the owner had paid for a number of fowls the dog had killed, and he had decided to have it "put to sleep."

I was soon to find out that the dog was a confirmed killer. We scoured the country for it but heard nothing more until the third morning after the escape.

I was then visited by a farmer client of my own, who stated he had found the dog in his poultry run where it had killed eighteen white Leghorn pullets he valued at twenty five shillings apiece. The dog had escaped after removing a piece from the leg of the farmer's trousers.

On the following morning there was a claim for seven birds

from three miles away, and after this, as the news of the lost dog got around, there were daily claims from every part of the country, with such distances between them that one could only imagine the dog had by some means acquired a bicycle.

At the cattle market next week, the master of the local foxhounds came up to me, shook me by the hand, and told me I was "a real pal." Ever since the dog had escaped he had remained quite free from claims for poultry killed by foxes.

I organised dog hunts but nobody actually *saw* the dog again until one day a farmer came to tell me that a dog, answering the description, was sleeping at night in one of his outhouses, in a field near the farm.

We laid down some saucers of food in the house doped sufficiently to produce sleep without being fatal. We expected then to have the dog at our mercy. During the next few nights my doped saucers accounted for seven chickens, two ducks, a cat and a greyhound, but still there was no sign of the Sealyham.

Nevertheless, the claims continued to mount.

One twilight evening I was standing under a cliff, rifle in hand, when on a rock twenty feet above me, silhouetted against the evening sky, I suddenly beheld the dog—motionless. I took careful aim at his heart, and was about to pull the trigger. But I got no further than that. The dog was so confident, so unsuspecting, such a perfect picture against the light of the setting sun. How could one take advantage of a sitting target? It seemed so unsportsmanlike. I laid the rifle against a rock and the dog vanished.

I offered a considerable reward for the dog, alive or dead. A fortnight later it was shot in broad daylight by a poacher.

The owner then made a serious attempt to sue me for the value of the dog. He failed, but I had to foot the bill for all the chickens that disappeared from that corner of the world throughout a good many weeks.

Chapter Nine

WHAT OF THE FUTURE?

NOBODY CAN GAINSAY the essential part which animals play in our national economy. They provide human food and human companionship—a curious association of ideas, not particularly in favour of the animal. They provide not only food, which includes milk, cheese and dairy products, but all the by-products other than meat and offal, in the form of hides, wool, leather, glue, bone meal, manure; and food material for other animals.

Animal husbandry and animal genetics constitute, today, an important part of veterinary science. Animals must be bred to provide the greatest quantity of human food, with a minimum of waste, and they must be bred in such a way that they carry the greater amount of meat on the parts from which meat is most expensive, with a minimum amount covering the bones of the parts where the meat is cheap.

Moreover, animals must be fitted with carcases which grow to killing weight in the shortest possible time at the lowest possible cost, and those animals which produce milk, rather than meat, must give the largest quantity in the season when milk is expensive, together with the maximum content of butter fat.

Residents of our cities and towns seldom realize, when they sit down to their "Sunday roast," when they put on their shoes or gloves, or settle down to knit while they watch T.V., what a vast organisation has been built up in rural areas to enable the townspeople to live. Wool does not grow on trees, butter has a long story behind it before is appears in the shop window, and beef does not walk into the butcher's shop.

They are produced only by human enterprise, much thought, a vast expenditure of capital, and a great deal of sweat and blood.

The people of Britain, whether they be factory workers, professional men, burglars or bishops, nearly all fail to realise that the wealth of the country lies not only in its factories, its mines and its shipyards, but in its people.

Its people cannot work without food. They are dependent very largely upon our home production of meat and dairy products, bread and vegetables.

They would have very little of these unless their country carried an efficient veterinary profession to maintain the animal population, and to keep animals in health. Without the animals and their manure, the public would have few vegetables, and little bread.

In fact the prosperity and the survival of any country in the civilised world is essentially dependent upon that basic requirement—food.

The food we eat is either of animal origin or it is grown upon land fertilised by animal products. The health, well-being, and prospect of survival of the human race is irrevocably linked up with the soil, and both the animals and the soil are directly or indirectly dependent upon veterinary science and veterinary service.

The factories and the shipyards are visible to every town dweller, but the farmyard, the fields, the bullock pens and cowsheds, are forgotten. If they come into mind at all, the average citizen visualizes them dimly, as spots where one treads very warily, holding a handkerchief to one's nose.

In addition to the fact that these creatures of the farm provide us with most of the necessities of life, without which we would starve, they also provide work and a livelihood for a considerable proportion of our population. Not only have animals to be tended and fed, but their own foodstuffs have to be grown and harvested, transported and distributed.

Even if you picture the muckyard as a dim vision of filth, which is brought closer to you only on some unfortunate occasion when you put your foot plumb into a sample, you should then remember that without a sufficiency of this admirable product, there would be no flour to make your pies and your bread; you would lunch without potatoes, cauliflower and peas; and breakfast without cereals, or even without bacon and eggs; for the creatures which provide these delectable foods, are also dependent as we are, upon the products of the soil. One cannot live on the output of the factories. Vacuum cleaners, refrigerators and washing machines are luxuries, but one cannot eat them.

The world is not dependent basically upon coal mines, upon roaring furnaces and the annual output of motor cars, but upon essentials, upon the herds in our fields, the sheep upon the hills and our yeomen on their farmsteads. Scorn them if you like; call them yokels and clodhoppers, disregard them if you will. But if you do so, tighten up your belts, for your stomach depends upon the sustenance provided by the skill of their brains and by the exercise of their labours.

Close down your factories for one week and the world will go on. Close down British agriculture for the same period and see what will happen.

So much for our food producing animals. How about our household pets, our dogs, our cats, our horses and ponies in the stables? Apart from the fact that without our cats, and to a lesser degree our dogs, the whole population would, in a short space of time, be at the mercy of a rodent plague, we must not be unmindful of the part which the companionship of animals in the houses exercises upon the psychology and social behaviour of the human race.

Satan ever finds mischief for idle hands to do, but idle hands cannot compare in this respect with empty hearts and frustrated emotions. The animal provides the safety valve in many a family.

The care of, and the love given to animals, keeps the individual not only happy and interested, but *contented in the home*. The dog by the fireside is a link, not only an outlet for affection, but a tie between members of a family, an interest which they share amicably. It is absurd to claim that the dog ever takes the place of the child in the home; birth rate is affected by a number of differing factors but one has yet to meet the couple who allowed the presence in the house of a Pekingese to influence in any way their private views, for or against becoming parents.

From their earliest historical records, animals have played a leading part in a great many of our national sports.

Many animals share the excitement of their human colleagues and are definitely exhilarated by human companionship. By the aid of human suggestion they can easily be persuaded to carry out all manner of daft antics, such as running round and round a circular track in pursuit of a plastic rabbit they have no hope of catching, and which would be of no use to them if they did.

Most human pastimes are equally futile, but as they expend energy which might otherwise be used up in more dangerous pursuits, there may be something to be said in their favour.

To assist in providing and maintaining the professional personnel required to keep the animal population at its required level, and to maintain its health and protect that of the human beings who associate with animals and eat their flesh and products, the profession is maintained under the aegis of two main organisations. The first of these is the Royal College of Veterinary Surgeons; the second the British Veterinary Association.

Until recent years, when all the veterinary schools were absorbed into the universities, the Royal College of Veterinary Surgeons acted as the examining body and undertook the registration of all graduates who, after a prescribed period of study, satisfied their examiners that they were suitable persons to act as members of the veterinary profession.

The course was long and arduous, and it has become even more so now that teaching is carried out in universities in place of the former veterinary schools. The new candidates for professional honours are all interviewed and hand-picked but the number of applicants is far in excess of the number which can be accepted and the list of young people awaiting admission is a long one.

Since the original "One Portal System" has been abolished, each university veterinary school now conducts its own teaching and its own examinations, but both the teaching and the examining are subject to scrutiny and approval by the Royal College of Veterinary Surgeons.

It is a little early yet to judge the final achievements of university teaching but up to the present it appears to have attained a high level of proficiency. The new university graduates have an excellent scientific background, probably unsurpassed by those of any other recognised profession. When I think of how little I, myself, knew when I obtained my diploma to practise, I cannot help thinking that the present day graduates enter into their new life with manifold advantages we "old-timers" never possessed.

They have opportunities to become acquainted with animal patients within the university schools to a limited degree, with excellent opportunity to practise surgery upon the dead animal, even if their 'live animal' surgery is wisely controlled.

But all students spend some part of their vacations in private practice under veterinary surgeons who act as extra-mural teachers.

While the Royal College of Veterinary Surgeons is the registering body and governs its members, the British Veterinary Association is devoted to the interests of the profession generally, but has no absolute control of professional activities. The Royal College retains its Disciplinary Committee and is responsible for the maintenance of professional integrity and dignity. This committee has power to remove from the Register of the College, the names of any of its members who transgress or bring indignity upon the College, and it may prevent them practising for a period, or altogether.

While the Royal College of Veterinary Surgeons is the registering and governing body, and the British Veterinary Association takes care of the interests of the members, the latter can only make suggestions and has no disciplinary powers.

The Association is composed of a number of divisions, many dependent upon geographical location, others representing groups of practitioners, such as those who teach and those who perform certain types of veterinary work.

Veterinary practice, unlike human medicine and surgery, is largely bound up with economics, excepting in small animal practice when the amount of treatment given will depend on the affection felt for the animal by its owner, and the amount of money he, or she, can afford to spend on its welfare.

There are charitable institutions which provide essential treatment for animals owned by people who are financially unable to pay veterinary fees. The number of such people today must necessarily be small.

Animals on farms, unless highly-bred, have a limited value, and as modern drugs, including antibiotics, are very expensive it is occasionally more economical to salvage the animals in some way, or slaughter them for food whenever the carcase is likely to pass the meat inspector for human consumption.

When animals are valuable a whole range of modern drugs, precisely the same as those used in human medicine, is available. As a bullock takes about sixteen times the human dose, the administration of costly antibiotics may be an expensive procedure. But, as in human medicine, the wide range of inexpensive drugs contained in the British Pharmacopoeia in now almost completely discarded, and one wonders sometimes whether medical and veterinary treatment carried out with their aid, until a very few years ago, was *quite* futile.

Fortunately, the modern tendency in veterinary practice is to charge a fee for mileage, time, skill and service, and to take only a nominal profit on expensive drugs.

Stocking a veterinary pharmacy, nowadays, is an expensive undertaking requiring much capital outlay, and it follows that now newly qualified assistants are in the £1,500 income group and expect a house and car to be provided, while some practices keep a large number of qualified assistants, the overheads have soared to tremendous heights and fees have had to rise proportionately.

A large part of the money paid to veterinary surgeons by clients goes into the funds of the pharmaceutical chemists, while the bulk of the remainder is used to run cars and keep assistants. As usual the poor principal gets the smallest share of the proceeds and the greatest share of the worry.

It is still to be regretted that Britain, out of all civilised countries, still permits meat at abattoirs, slaughtered or presented for human consumption, to be examined for soundness by lay inspectors instead of by qualified veterinary surgeons. This is not written with the intention of casting any reflection upon the existing meat inspectors who rely on their experience and are honest, painstaking people. There is no doubt, however, that it would be a great deal safer for the public if the services of the present meat inspectors were all subjected to qualified veterinary supervision.

Whatever the earlier generations of veterinary surgeons accomplished with their old-fashioned remedies, and a lack of knowledge (which the younger people engaged in intensive research are quickly remedying), it must be agreed that they retained and enhanced the prestige of their calling, and carried out their duties quite as capably as it was possible for them to do with the limited resources at their disposal.

But it must be remembered that in spite of their shortcomings (and those of this generation will be similarly lamented by the next), the knowledge they acquired and passed on to the present generation was not without value, since it was founded on practice and not upon theory.

It has formed the basis of present day knowledge, even if the younger people have added a deal more colour to the original picture.

In addition, the older school of veterinary surgeons forged a very strong link with their clientele. They were regarded as valuable counsellors, willing at all hours to give their services and advice. There was then in existence a practitioner-client relationship which possessed great merit—and is in great danger of being lost in this present go-ahead world, in which the lust for speed and wealth, have created a new set of values and a new code of living.

However socialistic the world may have become, and however satisfactory it may be to behold the erstwhile "labouring classes" revelling in luxurious, if not gracious living, those of us, who retain pleasant recollections of the bad old days, cannot escape feeling a twinge of regret that the atmosphere of the whole country now possesses so different an odour. The respect paid to those who owned the soil has departed, and the spirit of "I'm all right, Jack," has taken its place.

So far as veterinary practice is concerned, the old relationship between client and practitioner, the tie of mutual respect and liking, is becoming less evident. Even if it is still possible in certain practices to grow rich out of one's labour, something we failed to do in the old days, any feeling of satisfaction resulting from the fact is lessened by the knowledge that clients are not as they were.

The old camaraderie is missing and although the demand for veterinary service is greater than ever, it is because the majority of clients calculate one's service in terms of profit resulting therefrom; they have discovered that it is economically profitable to pay for veterinary advice.

Clients change their professional advisers for small reason or none at all, and to a great extent this has come about because the newly-rich client with no prior knowledge of animals has suddenly turned to farming or horse owning, or to breeding dogs, or Jersey cows, and possesses that small amount of knowledge which so often proves dangerous.

It is not only our own profession which suffers from this change in manners. It is a morbid condition which is general throughout society, more apparent to those who have lived and practised in more cultured days—among happier people.

Practices have changed too. The smaller single-handed practices have gone, and larger combinations carrying a number of partners and assistants, together with lay helpers, have taken their place.

Nationalisation would be difficult to operate and the prospect does not curry favour with the rank and file of the profession. In any case the land would need to be nationalised first.

Specialisation is common in large practices and each partner may associate himself, or herself, with some particular activity.

In some practices veterinary hospitals are becoming established, but for large animals the cost of keep and treatment in hospital is apt to be economically prohibitive, other than in research establishments and those maintained by public subscription.

Since every graduate now spends from five to six years in a university and receives a university degree, there will for a long time to come, be no dearth of applicants for admission. It is very important, therefore, that all intending entrants shall undergo careful "vetting" before being enrolled, in order that the profession may continue in the future, as it has in the past, to be composed of men and women who will uphold its prestige and bring honour to its ranks.